T0363548

Emotional Female
Yumiko Kadota

PENGUIN BOOKS

PENGUIN BOOKS

UK | USA | Canada | Ireland | Australia
India | New Zealand | South Africa | China

Penguin Books is part of the Penguin Random House group of companies
whose addresses can be found at global.penguinrandomhouse.com

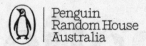

First published by Viking in 2021
This edition published by Penguin in 2022

Cover design by Yumiko Kadota and Louisa Maggio
© Penguin Random House Australia Pty Ltd
Internal design by Midland Typesetters, Australia
Typeset in 11.5/17.5 Sabon by Midland Typesetters, Australia

Printed and bound in Australia by Griffin Press, an accredited
ISO AS/NZS 14001 Environmental Management Systems printer

 A catalogue record for this
book is available from the
National Library of Australia

ISBN 978 1 76089 463 4

penguin.com.au

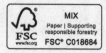

CONTENTS

For my sisters
Eriko and Mariko

A MESSAGE FROM YUMIKO

Hello. My name is Yumiko Kadota. I *was* a doctor. I *am* a doctor. I am . . . a *recovering* doctor. This book describes mainly my own experiences with mental health issues, racism, misogyny, bullying and sexual harassment. There are also references to others' experiences with sexual assault, domestic violence and suicide. As such, please do take care of *you* when reading this book, especially if any of these themes are triggering for you.

If you're in a toxic situation, I hope this book might give you the courage to leave, because you deserve better. Please know that nothing is more important than your physical and mental health.

Lastly, I am reclaiming the pejorative term *emotional*. If you've ever been called that before, I stand by you. Being emotional makes us human, and I'm certain that it made me a better doctor to my patients. Keep being emotional, it's a beautiful thing.

Lots of love,
Yumiko xx

PROLOGUE

March 2018, Sydney

I wake up just a few minutes before my alarm is due to go off at 5.41 am. My phone permits nine minutes of snoozing, which gives me until 5.50 if needed. Over the years I've learned that forty minutes gives me exactly the amount of time I need to get myself ready for the day. I go into autopilot mode. I lay the outfit I prepared the night before on my bed. I walk into the kitchen and turn on the coffee machine. While my coffee is being made, I grab the muesli from the pantry and some milk. I don't have time to sit down so I lean on a stepladder and eat over the sink. I haven't engaged in any sort of mindful eating in years, which is very un-Japanese of me. I swirl the coffee in my mug and add the milk from the frother. I never short-change myself with the froth. It's the only moment in the day that I can treat myself to something nice, before I make my dreaded way to the dysfunctional hospital that I've been calling my second home for the last few weeks.

It wasn't always like this. I've just come from a six-month rotation working at a children's hospital in which everything was shiny and cheerful for the kids. It was a state-of-the-art facility, attracting the best specialists. A place where I felt the drive to succeed and the heart to help. I left that term full of optimism for the year ahead. Two thousand and eighteen: it's going to be my year. It's been seven years of working towards what has become the career I most covet: that of a plastic surgeon. There are a few steps to take before I get there – namely getting selected for the advanced training program – but I am determined. Every cell in my body hungers for it and I'm trying desperately hard to keep up my enthusiasm. *C'mon, Yumiko, you can almost taste it.*

I carry the mug with me to my bed and for a split second I exhale and stare at my mirrored wardrobe. God, look at me. Since I started at this hospital, I've gained a considerable amount of weight. I stand with my belly hovering over the elastic of my underpants, wondering how I let myself go. I've been so disciplined throughout my career thus far, going to the gym every morning before work, and training on weekends. I used to have a spring in my step and an endless supply of energy. Now I'm exhausted, pining to get that bounce back. I miss exercise. I miss the feeling of my heart pounding against my throat and the rush of endorphins spurring me on. Most of all, I long for sleep, for a rest from the long, relentless days I am working.

I take a sip from my mug, staring blankly at my dull eyes in my bedroom mirror. Mid-sip, my phone rings to haul me back to reality. I look at it, resting on its wireless charging pad, absorbing the last few minutes of energy before we start our adventure together for a new day.

No Caller ID. The hospital. Startled, I place the mug quickly on the carpet, spilling coffee onto it, determined to answer the phone before it cuts off. Nothing is worse than missing a call from the hospital. It's most likely going to be a minor hand injury, which is the majority of my work, but there's always a possibility that it could be something life- or limb-threatening, when every second counts. Just in case it's the latter, I never want to miss a call. If I miss one, they might call my boss – the surgeon on call. And that's never a good look. Bracing myself, I make it on its third ring.

'Hello? Yumiko speaking.'

'Hello, is that Plastics?'

'Yes,' I answer. I'm used to being called 'Plastics'. No name needed.

'Oh hi. I have a man who accidentally hammered the top of his pinky and it's torn off half his nail.' I breathe a sigh of relief and my heart rate calms. My brain is a triage machine. This time, the category is 'not urgent'.

'Please get an X-ray make sure his tetanus shot is up to date and keep him fasted I'll see him after my ward round,' I say in one breath. It's a line I've delivered many a time before.

I finish my coffee, put on my clothes, and go to the bathroom to brush my teeth. I hear my phone ringing again in my bedroom. I quickly rinse out my mouth and run back.

'Hello? Yumiko speaking.'

'Hi. Plastics?'

'Yes. How can I help?' I look at my watch. At this time of day, I need fifty minutes to get to the hospital, find a parking spot, and start my ward rounds at 7.30 sharp. I have one minute to get down to my car in the basement. I'm itching to leave my apartment but the phone will cut off in the lift.

3

'Oh hi, how are you?' says a bubbly intern.

'I'm fine.'

'I was wondering if you can advise me on a patient. He had his tooth extracted yesterday and it's just started to bleed again. He's on blood thinners and I haven't been able to stop it.'

'The best way to stop any bleeding is by manual pressure. You have to press gauze firmly onto his tooth socket and hold down for at least seven minutes.'

'I have other patients to look after so I can't be there for that long with him. Could I get you to come and review him?'

A familiar sense of irritation creeps up like an insect crawling up my neck. The intern doesn't have time to hold a piece of gauze in her patient's mouth, so she wants me to do it instead? Because I have so much free time? I swat that insect and refocus.

'You can get the patient to apply the pressure. Check again in seven minutes and call me back if you have any problems.' I end the call and rush out my front door and into the lift.

The hospital rings again as the lift descends, but the ringtone gets swallowed by the underground. My heart is beating fast. I don't know whether it's because I've just missed a call or because the caffeine's kicked in. Probably a bit of both.

I hop into my car and wonder if whoever it was will call me back. I'm three minutes late and my heart sinks because I'm certain I won't find a parking spot close to the hospital now. I put the radio on – this is the only time during the day that I get to know anything of what's happening in the outside world, or at least what's in the Top 40. I'm driving when the phone rings again. Concentrating on navigating a serpentiform route towards the main road, I answer.

'Hello, is that Plastics?'

'Yes.'

'I called a while ago about a man with a bleeding tooth socket. It's still bleeding.'

'Have you tried soaking the gauze in adrenaline?'

'Umm, no.'

I take a breath. *Be nice.* 'Okay, well, why don't you try that? If it fails, you can inject some local anaesthetic with adrenaline into his gum.'

'I'm not comfortable doing that . . .'

I have to remind myself that I'm talking to an intern, and not all interns are as confident with doing procedures as I was back then.

'Do you have a registrar who can help you with the injection?' I ask.

'They're all really busy at the moment.'

'Okay, well, why don't you try the adrenaline-soaked gauze first, and if that doesn't work we can go from there. Can the patient follow up with his dentist today?'

'His dentist doesn't work on Tuesdays.'

I look outside my car window. I'm now several suburbs away from my cosy apartment on the leafy North Shore. It's less green, more grey. I drive past several used-car dealerships and factories. The landscape becomes increasingly industrial. When I finally get to the hospital, my resident, Kevin, and medical student, Thea, have the lists printed and are ready to go. Thankfully I don't get any more calls about the tooth socket.

'All right, team, we have a couple of consults to see in ED after our ward round – a man with a nail-bed injury, and a girl with a sore throat. Let's go!' I enthuse. I am the leader of the pack, I must keep the energy up. Kevin and Thea are always eager to help me, so I feel like I owe it to them to stay upbeat.

The first patient for our ward round, Mr Smyth, is not in his bed again. The nurses know what time we do the ward rounds, but always have trouble keeping him there. He's gone for his morning smoko. I'm going to have to find him later to check up on him. My pager goes off. It's the Emergency Department, probably wondering when I'm coming down.

The patient with the finger injury has a broken bone and will require an operation. Since it occurred at work, surgeons get well remunerated by Workers Compensation for such a procedure. However, I know the surgeon, my boss, will not be coming in. The long drive is not worth it – the surgeons would much rather be consulting in their plush city offices or operating at private hospitals. That's the thing about being a fully qualified surgeon. You might be appointed as a consultant in the public hospital, but the groundwork is done by people like me – the registrars. Private healthcare is different. The patient pays to see you – the specialist surgeon. So of course surgeons feel more inclined to give their time to their paying private patients. Why even bother having a public hospital appointment, then? I ask myself that all the time . . .

My fingers work faster than my brain and dial the operating theatre. Case booked. I recite my usual spiel to the patient: 'I've booked your operation and we aim to get it done this morning, but sometimes we have emergency cases that are urgent, so there's a possibility that your operation may be delayed, or if we're really unlucky it may not happen at all today and we may need to do it tomorrow.'

The patients always appear understanding when I deliver this well-rehearsed speech, until they get hangry at 10 pm and wonder why they're still waiting. Then, if they do get cancelled, they are both angry at being delayed and relieved that they now get to eat a stale sandwich and some cold custard from the hospital kitchen.

It's 8.30 am. I smile at Kevin and Thea and motion them towards the hospital café. We walk over there to collect the coffees and banana bread, which I've ordered on an app while we were in the Emergency Department. I'm constantly finding ways to save time in order to make more time for what's important, like the daily post-ward-round treat. The past hour has been spent making plans for fifteen patients or so, and I need to make sure that Kevin got everything down. I confirm the plans, explain how I'd like the tasks prioritised, and he carefully annotates his patient list with my order of importance. Then we enjoy some banana bread and banter.

A page comes in. HRH Sir Smyth has finished with his cigarettes and is ready for us to review his forearm wound. We head over to the ward via the operating theatre. The list is looking busy today.

Later, I go to the operating theatre to see if I can operate on my patient with the broken bone in his finger. I'm told that the nurses haven't had a lunch break yet, so theatres will resume in an hour. The General Surgery and Orthopaedics team booked a few cases after I did, and they categorised theirs as more urgent than mine so my surgery has been bumped to the end of the queue. I don't think I'm going to get it done today; it looks like I'll be delivering a few 'sorries'. Even though I'm fluent in the art of apologising to patients about delays, it never gets easier.

At 4 pm I let Kevin and Thea go home. The rostered hours for junior doctors are from 7.30 am to 4 pm, but Kevin and Thea always offer to stay back to help. They're good like that, but there's no point in holding them hostage at the hospital. BUZZ. My watch tells me I've gone past my ten thousand steps for the day. I must have walked to and from the operating theatre about ten times to check where I am on the list. With such little operating time available, I know everyone is playing dirty, manipulating urgency categories, and sweet-talking the nurse-in-charge to get their cases done. The other surgical specialties have consultant surgeons throwing their weight around in the mix, but I am powerless on my own. When you're performing operations as a lowly registrar, no one cares about placing you at the back of the list.

I go back to the registrars' office, and I wait, and I wait.

PART 1

Student

1

Decimal points

March 2005, Sydney

'Look at the person to your left. Now look at the person to your right. Two of you will fail medical school,' forewarned the dean of Medicine. It was orientation week at university and I sat in a lecture hall with 250 other first-year medical students. I had just finished high school at an all-girls school on the upper North Shore of Sydney. Being only one of two students from my school who were accepted into Medicine, I had high expectations of myself. But as medical students you are suddenly surrounded by people who were the top of their schools, so you know you might go from being the crème de la crème to getting creamed.

Flora was the other student from my school who'd made it into Medicine. She was my friendly competition through-out high school. She still resented me for coming first in her favourite subject, biology, but despite us being rivals, Flora was always supportive. Medicine doesn't have to be a zero-sum game. We can both be successful. Flora was living on campus and I envied her freedom as she got to roll out of bed five minutes before lectures. I knew I wasn't going to enjoy having to catch two buses to uni from where I lived with my family.

Throughout my schooling, both the left and right side of my brain were fostered, reflecting my dad's logical side and my mother's creative side. When it was time to apply for university degrees, it was between Music and Medicine. I chose my analytical left brain, much to the relief of my mother. Perhaps it reflected her own regret in choosing her right side. Yoshiko never had used her literature degree. Instead, she'd done what was expected of Japanese women at the time and become a stay-at-home mum.

There's a joke that Asian parents force their kids to study either Medicine or Law. That wasn't the case for me, but it was for Dad. Hajime wanted to study Mathematics or Philosophy, but they weren't acceptable options to my grandparents. Hajime always resented going to law school. He didn't enjoy it much, so he decided that he'd let my sisters and me do whichever subjects we wanted. I guess some would say he was 'lucky' that I chose Medicine on my own, fulfilling the Asian parents' dream.

That first day in the lecture hall, I looked up at the screen. It showed my path ahead as an image of a ladder representing the medical hierarchy. After six years of medical school, the first rung is an internship in a public teaching hospital, rotating between Emergency, Medical and Surgical terms. Next you become a resident, then a registrar, and finally a consultant in your chosen specialty.

Forms were passed around the lecture hall for us to fill out with some details about ourselves. I paused on the last question, which asked us what we wanted to specialise in. What do I want to be when I grow up? That was easy. Plastic and reconstructive surgeon. I remembered how I'd heard about surgeons reconstructing a man's injured jaw with a piece of his rib. How brilliant! Not only would it have been technically difficult, but the person who first saw the curvature of a rib and thought it approximated the curve of a mandible was a genius. Pure genius.

I looked around at my peers and wondered what they'd all written down. Surgery was considered cool but hardcore. Some of the other specialties were considered 'soft', like General Practice or Psychiatry. Paediatrics was for 'nice' people, because what kind of mean person would want to look after sick kids? The majority of people in the lecture hall were Asian – the model minority. I wondered how many were international students and how many were local. Even though I'd spent the last two years of high school in Sydney, I was technically an international student. That was something I preferred not to bring up, because it made me feel second class. I hated the stigma attached to it: some people at the uni thought international students were either rich kids who'd only been accepted into Medicine because Daddy was paying for it, or were bonded to their governments and so would be going back to their home countries after graduation. That meant we were perceived by some to be a waste of resources because we'd take our degrees 'home' rather than give back to the Australian healthcare system. Where was 'home' to me anyway? My family and I had left Japan when I was three months old and lived in the Philippines, Singapore and England before coming to Sydney. Australia was home to me now. Plus, I had worked so damned hard to get the required marks in my HSC and get on this course, and my parents were far from rich.

Wherever they came from, one thing was for sure, my fellow students were competitive. The first day of medical school had us comparing our University Admissions Index (UAI), which ranks students in the state. It was an inescapable conversation on the med lawn where we grazed between classes.

'What did you get?'

'.8. You?'

'Damn, I got .75.'

'I got .7, man.'

'Dude. what did you get?'

'.9.'

'Nice.'

Seriously. These guys were talking in decimal points, because they all got above 99. God save anyone who got 98.9! It was like they couldn't fathom anyone possibly getting a score below 99. Thank goodness I'd just scraped above that threshold. In previous years, I wouldn't have been accepted into Medicine because you had to get a UAI of 99.7 or above. The previous year, the university had changed the medical program. Medical educators around the world had realised that being knowledgeable was not enough to be a good doctor. A doctor must also be able to communicate effectively, to show empathy, compassion and humanity. While the old program was heavy on the sciences, the new program integrated other important subjects such as communication skills and medical ethics. After I graduated, they also started teaching students about burnout and stress management. To reflect this new direction, the entry requirements changed, too. Universities started introducing interviews and a test for logical reasoning, emotional intelligence, and non-verbal reasoning. My mother, Yoshiko, says I must've talked my way into Medicine. It's quite normal for Japanese parents to call their kids dumb. It's true that I was a talker, but they take modesty a little too far.

One person who definitely was not modest was Ralph. Ralph was a second-year medical student. That first day he was walking around the med lawn meeting the first years. You could tell that he enjoyed giving advice – he certainly had his two cents to share about every conversation topic that came up. Ralph was part of the old medical program, and should've been in third year. He told us that he didn't like the old program, which is why he'd abandoned it and re-enrolled in the new one. *Why would anyone want to repeat first year?* I thought. Ralph couldn't really explain to me what he didn't like about the old program, just that the new one was better. This was an unpopular opinion because a lot of old-school doctors criticised the new program for being too soft – there was too little time dedicated to the sciences. We were only the second cohort to start it. We were guinea pigs. A lot of my peers were concerned about this, but I wouldn't have known the difference between a good and bad medical education anyway – I was fresh out of high school. What would I know about what's needed to become a doctor? I was just happy to be there.

In many ways my mother was the perfect Japanese housewife. She would wake up every morning at 5 to cut carrots into the shape of cherry blossoms and turn apples into rabbits. I call my parents' marriage 'love by bento box'. One morning as she was making bento boxes, I was getting ready for my first tutorial at the hospital. In the past, students started clinical placements in fourth year, but as part of the new medical program we were to start going to the hospital once a week from first year.

Yoshiko scrutinised my polyester outfit from the corner of her eye and called out to me, 'You look like a waiter.'

'What?! How do I look like a waiter, Mum?'

'You're wearing a white shirt with black bottoms. That's what waiters wear.'

'But these are the only smart clothes I've got.'

'Are you going to ask patients whether they want still or sparkling?'

This was the kind of petty argument I'd have with my mother, who is well-meaning but harsh-hilarious. She was right, though, I did look like a waiter. To be fair, that's what I'd be doing as a medical student anyway: taking coffee orders for the doctors.

My outfit might have been synthetic but my excitement that morning was real. Despite her mockery of my outfit, I knew my mother was excited for me, too. Yoshiko handed both Hajime and me a bento box each. 'Have fun today,' she said, as she straightened my shirt collar, and then Dad's.

Bright purple lanyards with yellow 'Medicine 2010' logos adorned our necks as we entered a hospital for the first time as students. I wore my ID badge proudly; the only sign that I actually belonged in the health-care system. In all other ways we were pests in the hospital. There were six of us, including a girl called Lola from rural Queensland, whom I'd met during the Orientation Week. We bonded over the fact that we were seventeen, meaning we were missing out on a lot of the social events at uni, not that either of us was that interested in alcohol. Instead, Lola and I had coffee dates before our clinical tutorials. I'd only just started drinking coffee: a small sign that I was now adult-ing.

Hospital sessions were led by a clinical tutor, who could be any doctor at the hospital or in the community. Ours was Claudette, a GP from the Eastern Suburbs. We were taken to the ward to talk to a patient. A middle-aged man in a white gown sat in his bed with a paper in one hand. He peered over his glasses to stare at the six of us gathered politely around his bed. I was first up.

'Hello, Mr Lee. My name is Yumiko. I am a medical student,' I said awkwardly, peering up at Claudette for approval. It seemed my introduction was okay, so I continued. 'Could you please tell me what brought you to the hospital?'

'An ambulance,' he laughed while coughing at the same time, a glob of phlegm doing a flamenco in his airway. Ah. Probably something respiratory-related. 'I had a stomach ache that's been going on for a few days so I thought I'd get it checked out.'

'Oh. How would you describe that stomach pain?'

'Pretty damn sore.'

'Umm, where in your abdomen is it sore?'

'Kind of around here,' motioned Mr Lee, circling his entire abdomen.

'And do you also feel nauseous?' I asked.

'Nauseated, not nauseous!' interjected Claudette. 'Do you know the difference?'

17

'No,' I answered, feeling embarrassed.

'Nauseous means something that makes you feel sick. Nauseated means feeling sick. You must use the right words!' she said.

Mr Lee looked awkward while I was being told off, not sure where to look. I never used 'nauseous' again after that. I myself was starting to feel a bit nauseated, and I'd lost my line of thinking so Claudette moved me on. 'Okay, I might get Lola to take over from here,' she said.

I felt like I hadn't got a good go at this whole history-taking business. It was frustrating, but I retreated back to the group and quietly listened as Lola continued with the questions.

I left the tutorial feeling deflated. Taking a history was harder than I'd expected, especially in front of a group of peers and an intimidating tutor. I was determined to do better next time.

As the first week unfolded, I tried to become as involved as possible in extra-curricular activities offered on campus. Ralph encouraged all of us to audition for the Med Show, an original musical written by medical students each year. Ralph was a talented trombonist, and the music director for the Med Show. I'd just come off being the winning house music captain in Year 12, lifting the trophy for both the house choir competition as well as winning the overall music festival, so music was still high on my interests. There were several musicians in my year group. Again, the Asian stereotype was omnipresent – almost everyone I'd spoken to played either the piano or violin.

As an extrovert, I was equally interested in making friends as I was in becoming a doctor. I'd always thought that it was nice when someone you'd recently met addressed you by name, so I decided to memorise the names of the students in my year group. After the first two weeks, I could remember all 250 of them. Perhaps the nerdy part of me also got a kick out of memorising so many names. It reminded me of the game I used to play with my sisters to try to remember all the capital cities of the world. The effort seemed to be appreciated. Later that week, we had an election for first-year representative of the Medical Society, and I got voted in. I was on the council for Med Soc! Being a medical student wasn't enough for me: I didn't just want to do well at uni, I wanted to be liked, too.

2

The nail that sticks out gets hammered down

1982–1998, Japan to Singapore via the Philippines

My mother, Yoshiko, grew up in Tokyo, while Hajime was a country boy from Shikoku Island, in the south-west of Japan. When they met, Yoshiko had just finished her literature degree but work as a writer was hard to come by so she decided to find work in a bank, and it was there that she met my father. Hajime finished law school, but he never wanted to be a lawyer. He'd only studied it to keep his parents happy. He was interested in mathematics so it made sense to him to find a job involving numbers. He never expected it to be an easy nine-to-five at Mitsui Bank, but after a few years he found himself worn out from working 150 hours of overtime every month. In 1982 the bank offered a three-month conversational English program for its employees in an effort to improve international communications. *Stuff this*, he thought. *I'm going to enrol just to get a bit of a break*. It didn't take long before the program's instructors decided that Hajime's English was too advanced for the program, and so the bank instead sent him to the US to study a Masters of Business Administration – he even got a scholarship. That's when Hajime realised how big the world was and how much opportunity was out there.

My parents had only just met when Hajime won the scholarship, but he was keen to keep in touch with Yoshiko while he was away. Phone calls between America and Japan were expensive then, so they sent each other love letters. By the time Hajime returned to Tokyo two years later, he knew he wanted to marry Yoshiko. He was expected by his parents to marry a nice country girl from a respectable family but my father didn't care for other people's opinions, and in 1986 he and Yoshiko decided to elope: they got married in Hawaii, the Japanese people's paradise.

That year, Mitsui Bank was instructed by Japan's Ministry of Finance to send a capable employee to the Philippines to be seconded to and advise the Asian Development Bank – a financial institution established to help the economic growth of developing countries in the region. No one at Mitsui wanted to go. After two decades of corrupt and brutal dictatorship, President Ferdinand Marcos had been ousted and there was political unrest in the Philippines. Hajime, however, saw the role as an opportunity to do good, helping countries such as Sri Lanka, Bhutan, Nepal and Myanmar. He decided to take it on, and split his time between the Philippines and Japan.

I was born the following year in Tokyo, and after three months we moved to the Philippines, where Hajime was spending an increasing amount of time. My sister Eriko was born in 1989. A few months after that came the Tiananmen Square massacre, which sent seismic shocks around the world. At the time, Mitsui

21

Bank had a branch in Hong Kong but there were fears that China might repudiate the 'one country, two systems' agreement when the United Kingdom handed over sovereignty of Hong Kong, and Mitsui Bank decided it would be safer to pull out of Hong Kong and establish another branch elsewhere. They sent Hajime to Singapore to found a new merchant bank there.

That's how we ended up in Singapore, where I spent most of my childhood. When I was five, Mariko was born. Growing up, the three of us played together every day. We rode our bikes to the neighbourhood playground, which had a sandpit and a creaking seesaw. There was also a decaying treehouse made of old planks of wood with peeling paint. Mariko had a tricycle with pink streamers, while Eriko and I had bikes. Soon, we were reduced to one wheel – Yoshiko wanted us to experience some 'normal' things that Japanese kids do, so she got us unicycles. In 1989 the Ministry of Education in Japan had introduced unicycles to elementary schools, for children to build core strength and balance. It also taught perseverance, because, damn, that unicycle was hard to ride. I don't know how many times I fell off, but I never did master that particular skill.

Aya Ishikawa was my best childhood friend, and she lived down the road from us. Our neighbourhood was filled with Japanese expats who came and went every few years. We also knew families through the Japanese Association, where Yoshiko did some part-time administrative work. It was where our godmother, Hiroko Akuto, worked. Akuto-san was a religious woman. She treated me like her own daughter, giving me hugs when I needed them, each one like sinking into a plush cushion. It's not very Japanese to be affectionate and I never got hugs at home, so I treasured Akuto-san's.

I think we all craved a little more affection at home. I remember four-year-old Mariko coming home from kindergarten one day, tugging on my mother's skirt.

'Mummy,' she said. 'Hannah's mum calls her honey. Why don't you call *me* honey?'

'Oh.' This caught Yoshiko off guard. 'Do you want me to call you "honey"?'

'Yes.'

So our mother started calling Mariko 'honey' from then on, and sometimes 'darling'. It sounded strange and unnatural to my ears. I mean, it was in a Japanese accent, sure, but just the idea of it was weird. *Ha-nee. Daa-rin.* Who knew the Kadota household would ever hear such terms of endearment?

Akuto-san was a member of a new-age Japanese religion, Mahikari, and would often give us 'healing' sessions at our home, or sometimes we would go with her to the organisation's religious centre, called a dojo. Each session began the same way. We sat opposite each other, kneeling on the floor, Japanese-style. Bow twice. Clap three times. And then Akuto-san would chant a 'purification' prayer in ancient Japanese, and hold up her palm to radiate 'light'. If the 'receiver' had any ailments, she would cast her hand over that body part too. I wasn't really sure about all this 'light' business, but what I did like was that Akuto-san was selfless, caring, and dedicated so much of her time to healing others. Aya's mother also became a Mahikari.

Aya and most of the Japanese kids in our neighbourhood went to the Japanese school, but my parents wanted my sisters and me to have an English education so we were sent to an international school. We did, however, have a concurrent

Japanese education. From Year 1 to Year 8, Eriko and I studied the Japanese curriculum by correspondence. We had the same textbooks as the kids at the Japanese school, and every month a package with worksheets would arrive from Japan.

Even though I was growing up bilingually, English had quickly usurped Japanese as my first language. Japanese was difficult. Speaking it was okay because our parents spoke to us in Japanese at home, but the writing was challenging because we have three alphabets – *hiragana*, *katakana* and *kanji*, which is based on Chinese characters. On top of that, the verbs we use depend on who we're talking to – a system called *keigo*, which is divided into three levels of politeness. For Japanese people, physical gestures such as bowing, and language, are an important way of expressing respect and honour. So even if we're saying the same thing, the sentence is constructed differently depending on whether we're talking to a friend or someone higher up the social and family hierarchy, such as grandparents, a boss, or the emperor. If you don't use the correct *keigo*, you're considered rude and irreverent. Yoshiko gave us all drills and helped us, but it was frustratingly hard. She did not let us quit. '*Ganbari nasai*,' she would say. 'Keep going.' Begrudgingly, I would complete those worksheets and Yoshiko would post them to Japan. Teachers in Japan would mark them and post them back. We did this every month until I was fourteen and every month I'd ask, 'Mama, why do I have to do this? I already go to an English school. Why do I have to do Japanese school too?'

'*Sunao ni yarinasai*,' she'd say. 'Just do your work like a good, obedient child.'

Aya and I sang the iconic *Sailor Moon* theme song, which we knew off by heart, in Japanese.

'I'm Sailor Moon!' I'd announce.

'I'm Sailor Jupiter!' Eriko would chime in.

'I'm Sailor Venus!' joined Aya Ishikawa.

The Japanese language version would no doubt have horrified Westerners, who only knew the feminist, English adaptation. The Japanese lyrics open, '*Gomen-ne sunao janakute*' – 'I'm sorry for not being obedient.' Aya and I never discussed the meaning of the lyrics, though – we were too busy fighting evil. After playing sailors, we'd be off to our swimming lesson. Being just above the equator, it was a hot, humid summer's day every day in Singapore – the perfect place for swimming. Aya and I were very competitive. We would see who could hold their breath for the longest under water, as well as race each other. We had both started swimming lessons at the age of three. It was an expectation that all Japanese kids had at least one extra-curricular activity. Everyone belonged to a 'club'. Anyone who didn't have a club after school was seen as a loser. They were a member of the *kitakubu* – the 'go home club'. Who would want to go home? How boring. I wanted to try everything. Most days after school, I had somewhere to go. Every Monday, Yoshiko would take me to ballet classes at the YMCA. I'd started ballet when I was three, when I first wanted to become a ballerina. I continued until I was eight years old, when Monday afternoons were taken over by Brownies.

On other days, Eriko and I would go to the Japanese Association and Akuto-san would take us to the café for an ice-cream parfait. As we dunked our long-handled spoons into the layers of vanilla ice cream, chocolate fudge and crunchy cornflakes, we'd talk to Akuto-san about school and complain about our parents. Being the more outspoken one, I would represent

Eriko and myself as though we were plaintiffs in front of Judge Akuto. 'I don't understand why one education is not enough,' I'd say, and Eriko would nod along. 'Why must we also do the Japanese tests? The other kids get to play more than we do.'

At age four, I began playing the piano. Every day after school Yoshiko would make sure I played for an hour. She sat in a chair next to me and was strict about my practice. I always had to start warming up with scales. I hated scales. Yoshiko would explain that it was important to have good technique. I was never allowed to complain. If I was hungry or wanted to ride my bike, 'Gaman shinasai!' she'd say. 'Put up with it.' My sisters and I were all taught to 'gaman'. We were to do our homework and practise our instruments. Reward would come later. Both parents encouraged studying, but Yoshiko was the one dubbed kyoiku mama by the other Japanese mothers; a slightly derogatory term which translates as 'education mother' or tiger mum.

Hajime was big on giving everything a go. He took the role of my sports coach, and it was in this role that I felt I made him most proud. Whether it was sport or academia, Hajime always encouraged me to do whatever I wanted to. He didn't need to tell me that I had the tenacity to compete with any male – he already knew I had bigger balls than the boys around me, and I would be just fine.

As a nation, the Japanese are running-obsessed, and I was no different. The longer and harder the race, the better, and so it's no surprise that the Japanese love marathons. Marathon runners are national icons, and my role model was Yuko Arimori. I was seven years old when I watched Arimori win the bronze medal at the Atlanta Olympics. Four years prior to that, in Barcelona, she became the first Japanese woman to win a medal at the Olympics for the marathon, winning the silver just eight seconds behind the champion, Russia's Valentina Yegorova. Forty-two kilometres was an unfathomable distance. For me, 800 metres was long. That's the furthest we ran at school.

I was not interested in movie stars or singers. I looked up to athletes. In my eyes, Arimori was special because she was a female runner. Until those Olympics, I had really only watched male athletes such as the great Carl Lewis. At the start of each New Year my family gathered around the television to watch the Hakone Ekiden race. With a big expat community in Singapore, Japanese television was widely available, and I was glued to the screen as I watched the runners compete in the long-distance relay that took place over two days. The teams were from universities all over Japan, and the runners were men. There was intense focus on the athletes and coaches of each team, and this is where I first learned what hierarchy meant. The coach was the omniscient leader, never to be questioned. To keep harmony within the team, one must do as he instructed. This was the Japanese way.

My favourite part of the Ekiden was watching the steep inclines. There was something impressive about the uphill 'specialists', as they were called. The fastest uphill runners were lauded as 'kings of the mountain'. I liked the idea of being a specialist. I wanted to be a specialist in hills, too, which is what got me into cross-country running. We lived down the road from the Singapore Botanic Gardens, where Hajime would take me every week. I ran off the track, up and down the small hills. It was in these moments that I felt happy and free.

In 1997, aged ten, I travelled to Kuala Lumpur, Malaysia, to compete in a swimming and athletics competition with other kids from the Federation of British International Schools South-East Asia (FOBISSEA). Hajime was excited for me, and he accompanied me on the trip wearing the blue 'FOBISSEA' T-shirt like it was his favourite tee. He continued to wear it for years, well after its colour had faded. Hajime was a typical Japanese man in that he didn't show much affection. But whenever I saw him wear this T-shirt, I knew that he was proud of me, and it made me want to do well in sport.

At FOBISSEA I competed in butterfly and backstroke. I didn't want to swim front crawl like everyone else – again, I wanted to be a 'specialist', to stand out from the majority.

A few weeks later, back in Singapore, I competed in the Singapore Inter-Schools Track and Field Championships. I ran in the 100, 200, 400, and 800 metres, with my parents watching me from the concrete stands. We hadn't figured out what sort of runner I was yet, just that I loved to run, so my teacher let me run in all of the races. As I crouched down and placed my scraggy little fingers behind the white painted line, I could smell the rubber evaporating in the Singapore steam. I liked this smell, it felt special. It was not often that we got to run on a real athletics track. The smell and sounds from the stadium worked up quite a lather in me. They spurred me on to run so hard that I thought my legs would fly off my body. Still, my effort wasn't enough. I came close to last. The winner was a girl from Tanglin Trust School. Tanglin won everything. She was tall with long, powerful legs, and her shiny golden pony tail swung smugly from side to side.

What I learned from these races was that I was not a sprinter. I did a little bit better in the 800 metres. I realised that the longer distances were less about physical ability and more about willpower. As some of the other girls in my race started to tire, my inner voice told me that now was my chance. *C'mon, Yumiko, grip the ground!* I dug my spikes into the rubber and pushed forward. I still didn't come anywhere near the top three, but I was closer.

We also competed in field events. I was more 'track' than 'field' but I knew that some of the greatest runners were jumpers, too. Not many kids were interested in the triple jump, but I liked the choreography of it: hop, step, jump. Hop, step, jump! There was something satisfying about the syncopation of that rhythm. And, once again, I felt like triple jump was the 'specialist' event because of the fancy footwork. Channelling my best Carl Lewis vibes, I ran fearlessly towards the wooden board for my final attempt, not allowing myself to hesitate or slow down before take-off. Hop, step, jump. As I landed, I closed my eyes as the puff of sand created a snow globe around me. I stood up and looked back at the round pit my little bottom had made in the sand. It was good enough. I'd hopped, stepped and jumped my way to a bronze. It was the first medal I'd ever won in my life. I ran to Yoshiko with wide eyes and an even wider smile, leaving a trail of sand crumbs behind me. *Mama! Mama! I got a medal!*

I shared the podium with the Tanglin girls who'd won the gold and silver. For a small school that wasn't known for its athleticism (or much else, really), it was a big deal.

Winning the medal gave me confidence leading into the house captain elections in Year 6. I wanted to lead my house – in general, and certainly to more sporting victories. I wrote my speech and practised it in front of Eriko and Mariko, who formed my cheer squad. They sat cross-legged on the living room floor, as I stood up on the couch, much to my mother's dismay – 'Feet off the couch, Yumiko!' My sisters watched me recite my speech and clapped, even though Mariko was only four years old and didn't understand what I was doing. The actual speech went perfectly because I'd practised it so many times, and I got elected as captain of Cook, named after Captain Cook. Little did I know that I would end up in Australia six years later. The other houses were also named after explorers – Columbus (after Christopher), Hillary (after Edmund), and Armstrong (after Neil). As a quintessential Leo, I loved being the leader of my house. There was something about house activities that really stoked a fire in me. I loved the competition. I loved winning. But most of all I loved the feeling of belonging that being part of a house brought. The friends I had made through house activities had voted for me, and that approval felt great.

But with each feather on my little cap, hatred was multiplying. One hater's name was Agatha. Her dislike for me was like tiny fungal spores that propagated in the dirt. The more I succeeded, the more she detested me. She started to make fun of my academic interests. Being the *kyoiku mama* that she was, Yoshiko spoke often with my teacher. The mathematics was too easy for me. Because I had done the Japanese curriculum by correspondence, where the maths was harder, I was not challenged at school. So my teacher would send me home with advanced maths homework. I secretly loved this arrangement because I enjoyed maths. But, oh boy, when

Agatha found out, lunchtimes became unpleasant. Whenever I approached the girls' table, Agatha would whistle and the others would shuffle across the bench so that I would have no place to sit. I learned to eat quickly and find the boys in the playground for a game of soccer or basketball. As the saying goes in Japan, 'The nail that sticks out gets hammered down.'

The following year, some of the students from my primary school and I moved to the neighbouring secondary school. One night soon after I started there, I fell violently ill. We were out at a family dinner with the Ishikawas when I developed severe abdominal pain and started writhing on the ground.

'Yumiko! Get off the ground!' My mother was motioning me to get up.

'Mama, I can't! My tummy hurts so bad!'

As a lady who likes to keep up appearances, my mother was mortified that her child was on the filthy floor of a restaurant. Eventually my pain settled, but she took me to our family doctor the next day. The doctor was a skilful GP who was able to conduct ultrasounds. I suspect he'd been a specialist in Japan but having moved to Singapore had had to do what most migrants do, and enter general practice as his specialist qualifications would not have been recognised.

He scanned my abdomen and told me that my appendix was fine but he'd found a large tumour on one of my ovaries.

When our Mahikari friends were told my diagnosis, they prayed for me. They pleaded for me not to get surgery. 'Yumi-chan, I can't bear the idea of it. It reminds me of *harakiri*,'

Mrs Ishikawa would say, referring to the ancient Japanese tradition of samurai warriors stabbing a sword into their abdomens for dishonouring their families or, worse, their country.

Even at the age of eleven, I was strongly on the scientific side of the science–religion dichotomy. 'Mrs Ishikawa, I'm thankful for your prayers, but praying won't make this tumour go away. I need the surgery,' I said matter-of-factly.

My mother was a mess. One day after school I went to see Akuto-san and found Yoshiko there. She was on the floor, draped across Akuto-san's lap, sobbing into it.

'Come on, Yoshiko. Don't cry in front of Yumi-chan,' she said. '*Shikkari shite.*' 'Pull yourself together.'

I walked over to comfort my mother. 'Mama, I'm going to be fine. The surgeon said the tumour looked benign, remember?'

I wasn't nervous about going into surgery. To me it was simply something that needed to be done. Right up to the operation, Akuto-san continued to pray and 'purify' me. After her chanting I'd lie down and she'd cast her hand over my tummy to radiate 'light' onto my ovaries. Even though I knew the light wasn't shrinking the tumour, I still found the sessions comforting and therapeutic.

On the day of surgery, I remember being given the anaesthetic, counting down from ten to seven, and then waking up in the recovery ward. I stayed in the hospital for about a week. I quite liked being there – I enjoyed the care and attention I received from the nurses, and the food, even. My parents visited and Hajime would try to entertain me by telling jokes, but every time I laughed my abdomen hurt, so I begged him not to say anything funny. Typical Dad. He couldn't say anything tender, like 'How are you feeling? We're thinking of you. Are you okay?' but he was always cracking jokes. My teacher sent a teddy bear and a card, and I wrote her a letter back, thanking her.

Meanwhile at school, Agatha was spreading rumours that I grew a tumour because I ate too much. When I got discharged, she visited me at home with her mum, only to tell kids later how mangy my house was. I'd never thought of my family as poor, but when I found out she'd been saying mean things, and I thought about the houses the other kids lived in, I realised we did live in a simple unit.

I was apprehensive about going back to school after not being there for four weeks. My peers had all believed Agatha about my overeating, and thought it was funny because I was known for having a big appetite and I would always win fast-eating competitions. They'd call me a human garbage can.

I let them laugh about the tumour because I didn't want them to ask me where it came from: my ovary – gross. We were at the age when reproductive organs were still embarrassing to talk about.

Maybe Agatha did me a favour by telling tales about my tumour, but I still hated her. I also had some residual resentment from her bullying me in Year 6, so when I got the chance to yell at her for starting mean rumours, I thought of the worst possible swear words I knew at the time. I called her a 'fucking whore'. And that's how I got suspended.

I was so scared about what my father would say or do when he found out about my suspension. To my enormous relief it was Akuto-san who accompanied my mother to pick me up that day. I gave her a big hug. We all sat with the school principal, who suggested that my parents consider sending me to 'a stricter school for discipline. Perhaps an all-girls' school'. She told my mother, 'Yumiko will get in trouble for her mouth one day.'

3

'Your English is really good'

2001, London

During our time in Singapore Hajime was offered a few opportunities for work back in Japan, but as a family we'd always protested. My sisters and I loved our life in Singapore and didn't want to leave, especially not for Japan. Even though we looked Japanese – we were often reminded of that because people couldn't pronounce our names properly – we didn't always identify with Japanese culture. Besides, the resentment of having to complete Japanese education by correspondence put us off. Eventually, though, my father got a posting to London that he couldn't refuse. I was thirteen at the time.

So, in June 2001, the Kadota family left tropical Singapore – a degree above the equator – for London, fifty-one degrees north. My sisters and I had never been to Europe, and we were rather captivated by the thought of experiencing northern hemisphere seasons.

We travelled to the UK via Japan to visit our grandparents. First, our mother's side in Tokyo, and then to Shikoku Island.

Our grandma, Naoko, in Tokyo welcomed us home with her cooking. She made the best potato salads I'd ever known. She did this thing with hard-boiled eggs – crumbling the egg yolk over the salad as a garnish. That was my favourite bit. I loved how it made the potato salad look like a field of puffy dandelions.

The next morning, Grandma Naoko gathered us around the kitchen table and held up a spoon. 'Okay, little chickens, you each get one spoon and we will smash the egg shells.' My sisters and I looked at each other and smiled. We smashed them into little pieces, not knowing what it was for, but going for it anyway because it was fun.

'Now,' she said. 'We will paint the little pieces. You can choose any colour you like.'

We still weren't sure where this was headed, but followed her lead. After we finished painting, Grandma gave us each a piece of A3 paper.

'Now we each make a mosaic!' she announced. 'Use your imagination and create a picture using the coloured pieces.'

And just like that, Grandma Naoko got us creating art out of leftover egg shells from last night's dinner. She was an amazing woman. She always had ways of making something out of nothing. She'd led a simple life after the war and wanted to teach us that we didn't need much to have fun together.

After a week in Tokyo, we travelled south to Shikoku Island. June in Japan was humid, the hot air sticking to us like a flimsy shower curtain. The cicadas were complaining too. Even though I was getting a bit too old to be catching cicadas, being in Japan made me enjoy childhood pastimes. Our grandpa, Ji-chan, came with us to the local park. We carried nets and plastic cages, listening to the stridulations swarming around us.

'Look! Ji-chan! I caught one!' I yelled, running over to my grandfather with a large brown cicada in my net. Ji-chan laughed in delight. It was one of those wholesome chortles. 'Wow! What a catch, Yumi-chan!' he said, his bushy white eyebrows raised up high.

On the walk home, Ji-chan and I had our arms around each other's shoulders. I had a special bond with Ji-chan because we were both born in the Year of the Rabbit. Japanese people have a preoccupation with zodiac animals and the character traits they're associated with. Those born under the sign of the rabbit are thought to be sensitive, compassionate and have a strong memory. It was like Ji-chan and I had our own little club. Just us, the two rabbits.

The next day Ji-chan took us to the river for a swim – a very different experience from the barrenness of Singapore. I couldn't believe how clear the water was! My sisters and I lay on our backs, linking arms like a raft of otters. Summer in Shikoku was splendid. The sun was shining between huge candy floss clouds, the chorus of cicadas was as rambunctious as ever, and the stream was comfortably tepid like a daydream. Flanked between my sisters, I knew that life would always be okay because we had each other. We would be just fine starting our new lives in England.

After a few weeks in Japan, it was time for us to say goodbye to our grandparents and continue our journey. I wasn't scared or nervous. My sisters and I thought London was cool and we couldn't wait to discover our new city.

We arrived in London with sun-browned skin and matching goggle-tans on our faces. It was supposed to be 'summer' in

Britain but we were wearing cardigans. We settled right into the north-western suburb of Hendon, which was nicknamed the 'J-J community', so-called because there were lots of Japanese and Jewish families.

For the first time in our lives we lived in a house with a garden. Compared to the drab unit we'd had in Singapore, the house in Hendon felt palatial. Mariko and I shared a room, and Eriko got her own because she had trouble sleeping. Yoshiko was particularly excited about the roses and the lemon tree in the backyard. We spent the first few weeks exploring our neighbourhood and figuring things out, such as where we'd get the groceries. We found it strange that there was so much Indian food in England. Every supermarket seemed well stocked with microwave meals of chicken tikka masala. There was plenty of Indian food in Singapore, but Yoshiko cooked every day so we hadn't had much of it before. Imagine going to England to discover Indian food! I thought that was a bit funny.

We would be catching the Northern Line every day to go to school in the middle of London. I suspected my parents' choice of an all-girls school was influenced by my principal in Singapore, who thought I needed more discipline. Each morning we walked through an underground tunnel to get to Hendon Central tube station. The walls and ground were covered in graffiti and gum, and the stench of urine hit our little noses. Toto, we're not in Kansas anymore. The first time we went through this tunnel was when I realised how sheltered our lives on the sterile shores of Singapore had been. There, gum was prohibited by law, and the thought of anyone urinating in public was horrifying. We hadn't appreciated how clean Singapore was.

The school teachers met my sisters and me before the new school year began. The head of fifth form (Years 9 and 10), Mrs Higgins, was a plump woman with thick spectacles and hairs on her chin. I would be taking the British GCSE exams in two years' time, and she wanted to confirm my subjects with me. English, Science, Mathematics and a humanities subject were compulsory. I decided to continue learning French and Music for my elective subjects. I didn't want to take Japanese but Yoshiko and Mrs Higgins had decided it would be silly for me not to. I knew that as a fluent speaker I would find the subject too simple. I wanted to be challenged. I wanted to study something interesting. But Japanese would be a guaranteed 'A-star' grade. Besides, the teachers were concerned about my command of English, given that I'd come from this little island called Singapore. They were keen on selecting the right subjects for me to ensure the school would uphold its academic standing.

'I'd like to study Modern History as my humanities subject,' I said.

'Modern History is quite difficult,' replied Mrs Higgins, in deliberately slow English. 'You know, as you've come from Singgg-a-pore, you might find that you need to be quite good at English to study History. There's a lot of reading.'

I wanted to say, 'But English is my first language and I love Modern History!' but my parents were flanked on either side of me and I didn't want to talk back to my new teacher.

'Why don't you do Geography instead?' suggested Mrs Higgins. 'And perhaps Art as your other elective subject.'

'Yes, I think that's a very good idea,' agreed Yoshiko.

'Do you like Art?' asked Mrs Higgins, still speaking slowly at me.

'Yes, I love Art,' I replied quietly.

'Good, good. You don't really need to speak English for Art.'

I looked over at my sisters, who were as stunned as I was. I couldn't speak up. I wish I had told Mrs Higgins that the education system in Singapore was, in fact, quite excellent, and that the education there followed a British model. At moments like this I wished my parents had more guts. They were just so typically Japanese, too polite to contradict anyone. I actually didn't mind my final choice of subjects, but that wasn't the point. I hated the fact that I had been forced to forgo Modern History due to an assumed lack of English ability.

It took some time for me to prove myself at my new school. During my first week, the girls would say things like, 'Your English is so good!' They were lovely and well meaning, but by the end of that first week I was sick of telling everyone that people speak English in Singapore and that I had grown up speaking English just like them. They were all intrigued because most of them had never met a Japanese person. My sisters and I were the only Japanese people in my school. My sisters had some Chinese girls in their year groups, but I was the only Asian in mine. The girls treated us like dolls. They would touch my thick, straight hair, and compliment me on my cheekbones. I'd never even thought of my cheekbones before. I didn't know that they were 'high', and that high cheekbones were a good thing. Did they really think I was pretty, or were they just being nice? I wasn't sure. In Singapore, I didn't like that I was Japanese. I hated that my name was different. Westerners throughout my life would call me Yu-MEE-ko, but I never corrected them to say it was actually pronounced YOO-mi-ko because I was embarrassed. In fact, I'd say my own name the

'Western' way just to save the trouble. Sometimes I wondered whether it'd be easier if I just adopted an English name like some of the Chinese and Korean kids I'd met. But that would feel weird.

Midway through the first term there was a parent–teacher night that students were allowed to attend. I had achieved high marks in all of my subjects so I wasn't nervous. My grade for English was slightly lower than the others, though, so I was interested to see what my English teacher, Mrs McCown, would say. I sat next to Yoshiko as Mrs McCown told her that I was not 'naturally gifted' at English. Mrs McCown then turned to look at me with her steely grey eyes and said, 'You're not like Ruth or Clare. *Those* girls are gifted.' Those words hurt more than I was expecting them to. Mrs McCown looked a bit sorry for me as my eyes started to well up. Was she just saying this because I came over from Singapore? After that, I was even more determined to show her that I was good at English.

When the house debating competition came around, I put my hand up for it. I had never debated before, but I decided, *why not?*, thinking of my father's philosophy of saying yes to opportunity. It had been a good year for house activities. We had won the swimming, and now we were hyped up for the debating. Our team of three got through the early rounds easily and made it to the final, which was held in the assembly hall in front of the whole school. My heart was pounding with adrenaline. I'd always enjoyed public speaking, but debating in front of a whole school was next level.

The English style of debating was challenging, with girls from the other team shouting 'Point of information!' throughout my speech, which began to derail me. I wasn't used to being interrupted and having to think on the spot. After a while I started to shout back, 'Denied!' in an effort to try to keep to my arguments. It was lively and exhilarating. We ended up losing, but it felt good knowing that I had taken myself out of my comfort zone.

'Hey! You're so brave!' called out a girl in my geography class after the final.

'Oh, thanks,' I replied.

'I can't believe you just debated in front of the whole school. I can't imagine doing that in another language,' she said.

It didn't take long for me to feel like I'd fully assimilated into London life. I had my Northern Line friends who caught the tube with me every day. My friend Lou lived in Golders Green, just two stops before mine, so sometimes I'd get off at her station and we'd go to a café after school. Other days we'd go to Brent Cross, between our two stations, to the shopping centre there. Naturally, I found myself making friends through sport. There were just three of us in the swim squad – Nikki, Catherine and me. I was also on the water polo, rounders and basketball teams, but swimming was my favourite. I was feeling confident academically, too. Mrs McCown wasn't going to stop me from reaching for the stars. When the opportunity to apply for scholarships for sixth form came about, I applied for both academic and music scholarships. I wasn't sure yet what I'd do in the future. I knew that I had a creative streak but I also loved maths and science. There was an exam and interview for the academic scholarship, and for my music audition I played a Chopin étude on the piano. The following week I was awarded both scholarships, and in that moment I felt like I had finally proved myself at the school.

However, I didn't get to live out my final two years there as a scholar because Hajime got a transfer to Sydney. I couldn't believe it. Why so soon? I felt like I'd barely got to enjoy London. I loved it and didn't want to uproot my whole new life to move yet again. I'd have to get used to a new school and make new friends. The thought was crushing.

Uncertain about the quality of education in Australia, my teachers argued with my parents about keeping me in London. A few of them even offered to host me in their homes, but my parents were adamant that they wanted to keep our family together. I was furious with them. Why were they robbing me of this? I got *two* scholarships! Each year, several of the graduating class were accepted into either Oxford or Cambridge universities. During my time in London, I had romanticised about going to Oxford, and being awarded the scholarships had made that daydream seem a bit more realistic. But no. My parents were not engaging in any conversations about me staying. I suspected it was to do with 'discipline'. Ever since I'd been suspended from school in Singapore I felt as though I could never shake off the 'bad kid' label. They didn't trust me to live under a comparatively libertarian Londoner's supervision. I don't know what they were afraid of. Drugs? Alcohol? Sex? Probably all of the above. And so my parents continued to have a stranglehold on me and we were off to Australia.

My sisters and I didn't know much about the Land Down Under. Our only impression of Australia was the massive poster of *Home and Away* plastered on the wall opposite the Northern Line platform at Moorgate station. I'd never watched an episode, but I imagined it consisted mainly of tanned blonds walking around with surfboards.

It had been a short eighteen months in London, yet that time was transformative. I'd gone from a small country like Singapore, just a dot on the world map, to a major metropolitan city. That did give me confidence that I could move anywhere in the world, make new friends and start a new life. The scholarships gave me confidence in my abilities, even if they'd been doubted when I arrived. I reflected on how I was first treated. Would I have to prove myself everywhere I went because of how I looked? Now that I'd done nearly two years of study in England, would people just accept that I could speak English properly when I got to Sydney? I wondered whether I would end up being the only Asian in my year group once more. Living in London had made me feel different for the first time, in both a good and bad way.

4

Shameful secrets and invisible illnesses

At the start of my second year at uni I was organising Med Camp – a weekend away to welcome the first years. I was so excited to meet the freshers and tell them how great Medicine was! I'd loved my first year of medical school, and I was enjoying the first few days of second year, too. We were learning about the brain. It was complex and fascinating. I especially loved learning about the limbic lobe – the centre for emotion. It is intimately associated with other brain functions, which explains why we have feelings when we process physical sensations. Smell and fear. Pain and suffering. Memories and nostalgia.

I have known I am emotional since I was a little girl. I remember crying in an assembly when I was ten years old: the principal had told us that the man who worked in the cafeteria had been fatally hit by a car outside the school. I immediately began to sob. The kids in the row in front of me turned around to stare. I couldn't help it – I felt so sad for him. He was an elderly man with a hearing impairment. He didn't talk, but he always waved and smiled at us. *What an awful way to die,* I thought. I pictured him walking out of the school gates and a vehicle running into him. I guess he wouldn't have heard it coming. I imagined the shock he must have felt when he got hit, the pain and horror of it. I wondered whether he got killed instantly, or if he'd suffered for a while. Poor Mr Cafeteria Man. I went to the Japanese Association after school and told Akuto-san about it. She gave me one of her hugs.

I was sensitive in the true sense of the word – very responsive to all five senses. I remember practising for my flute exam when I was twelve years old. My teacher ran me through some aural tests.

'I will play two passages,' he said. 'Tell me what is different.'

He played them on the piano.

'Instead of playing C,' I reported back, 'you went up to E the second time.'

He stared back in disbelief, and stood up from his chair. 'You've got perfect pitch!'

'What's that?' I asked.

He sat back down and played an F sharp. 'What note did I play?' he asked.

'F sharp.'

B flat. G. C sharp. E flat. It continued. Whenever notes were played, I heard the name of the note as well as its sound. I'll try to explain. When I first started learning the piano, my teacher would sing the notes 'do-re-mi' along to my playing, so I learned to associate sounds with their names.

So, whenever I hear a tone now, I hear its name at the same time. But I didn't know it was called 'perfect pitch'. It's just the way my brain worked.

It was interesting to learn about parts of the brain like the hippocampus, too. It's part of the limbic lobe and is responsible for short-term memory. It also connects sensations and emotions to memories, such as when the smell of certain foods takes you back to childhood. I knew early on in medical school that having a good memory was an advantage, because I didn't have to study as hard as some of my fellow students. I knew the key to this was to concentrate in the first place, not just listening to what the lecturer was saying but paying attention to all of my senses. I was always fully present. I would sit in a lecture hall, remember who was sitting to my left and to my right. I could picture the slides projected on the screen inside the auditorium. The diagrams. The colours. What the lecturer was wearing, the sound of his or her voice, particularly if there was a distinct accent. The smell of the coffee I'd place on the plastic table that swung up from the side of the chair. All the senses. By doing this, I knew I'd free up time to do all my extracurriculars rather than having to study.

One day in the second term I had just attended a neuroanatomy class taken by our lecturer, Dr Norman, and was feeling inspired and thrilled all over again to have made this course. I loved anatomy. It was my favourite subject, partly because I was a visual learner. Some of the other subjects like physiology were more conceptual. For me, seeing is believing. I wanted to learn more, and always had questions after class. Dr Norman had another class to go to, so we walked and talked at the same time. She looked across the med lawn and squinted. 'Is that Ralph?' she asked.

'Yup, looks like him,' I replied, spotting Ralph on the lawn with the directors and producers from Med Show.

'What's he still doing here?' she said, rolling her eyes.

'What do you mean?' I asked, confused.

'He kept failing last year. Why's he hanging out on the med lawn?'

'He did?' I gasped. 'He's doing Med Show again this year so he's probably waiting for an Exec meeting . . .'

As my words trailed off, I realised what Ralph was doing. He was pretending that he was still enrolled in Medicine. Confident Ralph. It was all a façade. I suddenly felt sorry for him. He hadn't been coming to the lectures and practicals on the brain and he'd told us it was because he needed to help at his father's business. I guess he was still involved in Med Show so that he had one last connection to Medicine. I wondered how long he was going to keep this up for. Eventually Ralph stopped coming to university and no one heard from him after that.

That afternoon I met up with Bill, the president, and Dean, the treasurer of the Medical Society. As the outgoing first-year rep, it was my responsibility to organise this year's Med Camp, and I needed to finalise the plans with them. Bill was a tall and broad guy, whose physicality meant that he could easily command anyone's attention – I guess people like that get naturally selected into leadership roles. Being a small girl, I always felt I had to try harder with my personality and enthusiasm. Bill was now in fifth year. I wondered whether he was top of the class, as well as being top of the social hierarchy. Everyone in the years above me seemed really smart, so I wouldn't have been able to guess. I was determined to do well in both my studies as well as in Med Soc. The treasurer, Dean, was quite a flirtatious character, which made discussing the budget a little distracting. He eventually became my first and only boyfriend at medical school, but not for long. Dean was obsessed with money. I suppose that's what made him a great treasurer. In his spare time he would read books and attend business seminars about how to become rich. He said surgeons made lots of money; he wanted to become an ear, nose and throat surgeon. While we were going out, increasingly his attitude to money and medicine put me off him. I thought people entered medical school because they wanted to help the sick.

Around May that year Dean became ill with glandular fever and gave it to me. I contracted it more severely, developing chronic fatigue. I remembered a few kids at school getting chronic fatigue. It was a mysterious illness to pretty well everyone, and that certainly included Yoshiko.

'C'mon, Yumiko, go to uni,' she'd say, pulling the covers off me.

But I simply was not able to get up on many mornings. I felt continually exhausted.

'You're going to get behind in your studies,' she'd say in a pressing voice.

'You don't understand!' I cried. 'I'm so tired I can't even walk to the bus stop.'

Yoshiko knew I would never pretend to be sick, so she was worried as well as frustrated. I guess it was hard for her not understanding what I was going through but I resented her for not getting it. I felt as if my body were a formless, lifeless blob on the bed. The fatigue invaded all my muscles, and it frightened me. This was not me – I was supposed to be an energetic person.

It soon started to affect my friendships. I loved working with a buddy of mine, Neil. Choosing team members for a group project was like picking sports teams at school, and he and I would always pick each other first, as the strongest players. We knew that if we were both on the project together, we would get a good grade. This term we had a group assignment on the Gardasil vaccine. It was one of the big news items for 2006, a vaccine against the human papillomavirus strains causing cervical cancer had been developed and would be rolled out at schools all over Australia. A vaccine to prevent cancer. To me, this was incredible. What a monumental achievement for science, and public health. And yet I couldn't get excited about this project because I felt so drained fighting my own virus.

I could barely ever make the meetings, but I asked Neil to let me know what needed to be done and I promised I would do it. My group members knew that I'd had glandular fever, but that was a few weeks before, and though I tried to explain what was wrong with me, they couldn't understand why I was still at home. I wished I were walking around with crutches and a cast on my leg, or had a big bandage on my head. Chronic fatigue was a vague diagnosis that a lot of medical people didn't take seriously, and it was an invisible illness. I was tired – that's all I could say, and it seemed like a weak excuse. Neil felt he was the one doing the heavy lifting – he never said anything to me directly but one day I overheard him talking. I had just returned to university after several weeks of not being able to get out of bed and there he was complaining to a first year about how useless I was for the project. I'd never been a confrontational person but Neil was supposed to be my friend. I was fuming and on the verge of tears. I waited until he was alone before launching into him.

'Useless! If you have a problem, why don't you just tell it to my face?' I asked him, furious, and surprised by how upset I sounded. 'You're supposed to be my friend! I've been sick!'

'I'm sorry,' he said, a lurid hue of red spreading across his face and down his neck.

I glared straight into his eyes – I had nothing else to say. It was a horrible moment: I felt used, and wondered if all of my friendships in Medicine were going to be this fickle. It was hard enough battling this lingering, unyielding fatigue, without being treated like that by a friend.

I didn't have time to dwell on it, though, because at the end of the first semester, which was a few weeks away, we had exams. The faculty wasn't that helpful. They did at least say that if I were to fail one of the exams they would let me resit it because, they acknowledged, I was sick. That wasn't an option for me. I wasn't going to let myself fail in the first place.

Being the *kyoiku mama* that she was, Yoshiko was keen to do everything she could to help me. She wasn't the most confident driver, but she gave me a lift whenever I was too tired to catch buses to and from the university campus.

As I felt the strain of learning everything that I had missed in the preceding six weeks, I wondered whether this was a sign. Did I get sick for a reason? Was the universe telling me that I did too much? I knuckled down and studied feverishly for two weeks. Yoshiko gave me all the encouragement that she could. *Don't worry, Yumiko. You're strong when it's critical*. It was true. I always seemed to do well under pressure. That term, I got a high distinction at the exam. I didn't tell anyone, of course.

5

Biological creep

2007, Sydney

Surgery! Finally. I was so excited to be going to the operating theatre for the first time. It had taken me the rest of my second year – a good six months – to regain my energy, but by Christmas it was back. I didn't do anything in particular. I guess I just got on with it, and as the fatigue gradually disappeared my enthusiasm for Medicine returned.

It was the first term of the third year, which was divided into five eight-week blocks across the various specialties. My friend Matt and I were doing our clinical placement at the Children's Hospital. Our supervisor was Dr Little, a paediatric surgeon. He was lovely to his patients and their parents, and to us.

Matt and I were both crazy about the prospect of becoming surgeons, and we didn't waste time in expressing our keenness to Dr Little. He smiled and started quizzing us, first about the specialties we were interested in. For Matt, being a tall bloke, Dr Little guessed orthopaedics. And then for me . . . paediatric surgery? We both nodded. Matt was indeed keen on orthopae-dics, which was a popular specialty. It was seen as a masculine one: it requires brawn for sawing bones and hammering nails. I still desperately wanted to do plastic and reconstructive surgery but I wasn't going to contradict Dr Little. (I did end up loving paediatric surgery, but not quite enough to stop me pursuing plastics.)

This placement was the first time I got to see plastic surgeons work in real life. I learned about tissue expanders – balloons placed under the skin to stretch and create more skin for kids who have large lesions that need removing. I was in awe of the magical properties of the skin, how it could stretch and move to fill in the gaps left behind. I studied mechanical and biological 'creep' – the effect of stretching the skin with chronic force, like when pregnant bellies stretch to accommodate a growing baby.

One day I followed a plastic surgery fellow to the oper-ating theatre. He was using some cartilage in a little boy's ear to reconstruct his eyelid – how fascinating! He allowed me to scrub in for the case. I was so excited and went to the scrub bay to start washing my hands. A nurse followed me, her hawk eyes scrutinised the soap suds on my arms. Without saying a word, she re-entered the operating theatre to tell the surgeon that I was not scrubbing my hands using the correct technique, and instead of teaching me how to do it properly they decided that I should sit out of this surgery. My heart sank. Why couldn't she just have taught me the technique? I walked back inside with my proverbial tail between my legs. I tried not to look disappointed and still asked questions to seem interested.

'Did you know that if you put ear cartilage in the eyelid, the eye will start to hear?' he asked.

'Oh really?' I responded in disbelief.

'No, of course not!' The room erupted in laughter. He may as well have added 'you idiot' at the end of his sentence.

'How silly of me,' I said, embarrassed.

'Don't worry about it,' he said, and proceeded with the rest of the surgery without talking to me, so I left the operating theatre feeling dumb.

Days like these stood out because they were uncommon. Most of the time I went home beaming because I'd learned something new, or seen something interesting at the hospital. I didn't want to tell my parents or sisters about the embarrassing days or the sad ones because I knew they'd be upset.

One person I would have confided in was Akuto-san. A few years prior, in 2003, we had gone back to Japan to visit friends and family. As soon as we arrived at Grandma's place in Tokyo, my mother received a call from our old friend, Mrs Ishikawa. My mother's voice immediately changed. There were a few gasps. 'Akuto-san?' yelped Yoshiko. I knew before she hung up the phone that Akuto-san was gone. She had died during our flight over. It turned out that she had developed cervical cancer a year earlier but my parents hadn't told us because they didn't think she was going to die. In their eyes, Akuto-san was invincible. As a devoted member of the Mahikari religion, she was always the one 'healing' others. How can the healer become the patient?

That week, we went to her funeral. I broke down uncontrollably after I saw her body in the casket. I couldn't believe she was gone. Could she really be? Selfishly, I still needed her in my life. Who would hug me now? I had never seen a dead body before, and seeing her lifeless, ice-white face drained the warmth from mine. None of our other family friends was crying. Why wasn't anyone crying? Why was I the only one who was distraught about this?

After the ceremony, we went to dinner with two other families we'd known since our Singapore days – the Ishikawas and the Nishimuras. They were sharing stories about how wonderful Akuto-san was, and laughing over the funny memories, but I found it impossible to join in. I didn't want to eat. I wanted to leave this celebration of her life and cry. I knew they were in a cheerful mood because that's how Akuto-san would have wanted them to be, but still I found it hard to observe. Why couldn't we mourn just for one second? Japanese people don't tend to show their emotions, and I felt as though a metaphorical muzzle had been placed on my face, but I was too embarrassed to talk to anyone about how I felt about losing her. I never got a chance to share my grief with anyone. Life went on, and no one spoke about her death again.

I started a new rotation in oncology in mid-2007. Our orientation included a tour, which came to an abrupt halt when we got to the chemotherapy section. That's when I started to cry and couldn't finish the orientation. Memories of Akuto-san came flooding back. How stupid she was to think her faith could overcome cancer! I suddenly became angry. Why didn't my parents tell me when she'd been diagnosed? Why doesn't Japan have a public health screening program for cervical cancer? She didn't have to die.

The registrar who was taking the tour didn't know what to do with a crying student, while the other students stood staring at him wanting to continue with the tour. After a bit of hesitation, he told me to sit out the rest of the orientation and brought me to see his boss, Professor Dubia. Prof Dubia was a softly spoken man with spectacles as thick as magnifying glasses. He asked me about Akuto-san. He referred to her as 'Hiroko', which took me aback. We never referred to our elders by their first name, especially if they've passed. Dropping the suffix is called *yobisute*, which translates to 'call and trash'. It was highly offensive. I knew that he wouldn't have known that, but it still bothered me at how casually he was referring to my late godmother.

After I'd told Professor Dubia about Akuto-san, he asked about my past romantic relationships and then about my relationship with my father. These questions came out of left field and they made me feel uneasy but, not wanting to offend him, I answered him honestly: that all I'd ever experienced was my short relationship with Dean; and that my father wasn't particularly affectionate. Prof Dubia then explained that he was a trained counsellor and asked me if I'd like a session with him. Taken aback I accepted, surprised that someone as senior as him would be so kind as to offer support to a student. He asked some other personal questions, including my birthday, which happened to be coming up. I figured that this was his way of building rapport with me.

On my birthday an enormous bouquet, nearly as tall as I was, arrived for me. Later that afternoon Prof Dubia found me on the ward and asked if I had received the flowers.

'Yes,' I replied. 'Thank you so much. I was amazed. No one's ever given me flowers before.'

'I didn't think so,' he said. 'I was interested to see how you'd respond.'

I thought this was a bit of an odd thing to say. So the flowers were some sort of psychological experiment? Perhaps he came to this idea because of the conversation we'd had about men.

'You can't possibly travel on the train with those – let me give you a lift home,' he offered. I accepted the ride. He suggested that we go to dinner at a local Thai restaurant near the hospital that he wanted to try out. He must have seen the hesitation on my face because he added that my friend Belinda could also come along.

I kept going to Prof Dubia's counselling sessions, thinking that I should really get the support I'd needed at the time of Akuto-san's death. I wanted to perform highly in oncology and I knew that carrying around unprocessed grief would stop me from moving on and potentially impact my ability to learn.

During one counselling session, which took place after I'd finished my placement hours, Prof Dubia said he would close the door for privacy and asked if he could turn off the lights so that I could close my eyes and do a meditative exercise. I sat in his armchair and tried to get comfortable. He told me to breathe. He stood behind the chair and started touching my ears. 'Does this feel nice?' he asked. It didn't, but I said 'yes' out of politeness. I knew something was wrong. Fear spread like ink on a tissue. I froze, not knowing how to get out of the situation. He was slowly testing me by starting somewhere that wasn't overtly sexual and working his way towards my chest. It was when the back of his hand stroked my chest that my fight-or-flight response finally kicked in.

'Oh, look at the time. I really must go to catch my train,' I said as I stood up frantically from the armchair.

'Can I give you a hug?' he asked.

'Sure,' I said, not thinking much of a hug. When he hugged me, he untucked my blouse from my trousers and placed his cold hands beneath my blouse, on the small of my back. I lunged backwards, grabbed my bag, and ran to the train station. What just happened? My skin felt hot and prickly. I felt disgusting. That was the last time I ever went for counselling.

I couldn't believe how naïve I had been. But I was also deeply shocked that someone as well-respected and seemingly gentle-natured as Professor Dubia would behave like this to a student, or to anyone.

When I got home that day I called my friend Lola straight away.

'Oh honey, I'm so sorry,' she said. Instantly I was relieved I'd called her. Lola's soft voice was always such a comfort to me.

'What do I do?' I asked her, genuinely torn.

'I think you should tell someone.'

'Really? But I don't want to get into trouble.'

'Miko, why would *you* get into trouble? He's the one who did the wrong thing.'

'Well, yes, I know, but what if he finds out? What if he ends up being an examiner and fails me or something?'

'You shouldn't worry about that. You need to tell someone at the uni so that he doesn't do it to anyone else,' said Lola, this time in a much firmer voice.

She was right. I didn't want him creeping on other girls and I knew he shouldn't get away with treating me or anyone else like he had. So the next morning, I contacted a faculty member to tell her what had happened. Dr Fern Walker was in charge of student wellbeing. Her office smelled of incense and had an old fabric couch and lots of photos of her cats on the walls. She was wearing a dress with sunflowers, and some gold-framed glasses. She asked me if I wanted to make a formal complaint. I thought about it for a moment and decided that that seemed too over-the-top. I felt like there was some sort of shame that came with being a victim, but I hated that I was the one feeling shame when I'd done nothing wrong. It was an icky, slimy feeling.

I felt slightly less alone after talking to Fern. I didn't want to tell my family because they would be devastated, and apart from Lola I certainly wasn't going to tell any other students. I was also worried that I'd be criticised for putting myself into that situation in the first place. Would I get asked what I was doing in his office after hours? Would they think I was asking for it?

Fern was warm and empathetic, but kept an air of profes-sionalism. Honestly, I wished she'd just come out of her faculty role and say 'What an absolute creep! We need to get rid of him!' And I wished she would tell me what I should do. I wanted her to be firm and say we should definitely report him and that the uni would dismiss him or at least issue him a warning. But I knew she couldn't. 'It's up to you,' she said. I really wished it weren't. I was already embarrassed about talking about what had happened, so I didn't want to involve more people than was necessary.

Eventually Fern and I decided that she would inform the head of my clinical school because I was concerned that

Prof Dubia might have behaved in the same way to others in the past, and that he might do it again. Fern assured me that she would keep my complaint anonymous.

Luckily, my oncology term was about to finish and I would move on to palliative care at another facility. But I kept wondering how I'd let it happen. How had I been so unaware? Prof Dubia was a talented teacher, and I had benefited from his teaching, but I could see how that was his currency to lure me in. Sure enough, I got emails from him offering help for exam preparation in the following weeks. It sickened me that he thought he could try again. His audacity and arrogance filled me with fury. Not today, Satan. I was clamped between anger and helplessness. I wanted him to be accountable for what he'd done, and to be punished for the assault, but at the same time I was terrified of putting my future career at risk before it'd even started.

6

Room 101

2008, Tokyo

In January 2008 my grandfather Hiroshi died, my mum's dad. He was at home in Tokyo, with my grandma, Naoko, by his side: she had been his carer for the last few months of his battle with colorectal cancer. My grandfather became the classic picture of 'cachexia', which I'd studied at uni – someone whose disease had eaten away their bodies. It's medically described as looking 'wasted'. What a horrid description. My grandfather, bedridden in his last days, was just a skeleton draped with crepe-thin skin. He was too tired to talk and could barely get any words out towards the end of his life, which was disturbing for someone who had spent his life as a journalist for a Japanese newspaper.

Doctors were worried about my grandma being able to look after my grandfather on her own, but she was determined to do so. There was no way she was going to allow anyone to put him in a palliative care facility. She was a loving and devoted wife, and did everything to make my grandfather comfortable. She even rented a hospital bed to put in their tiny Tokyo flat so that she could move him in and out of bed more easily, and, using its remote control, sit him up for meals. She made sure he wasn't developing any pressure sores, following a tight 'turning' schedule to ensure he wasn't lying on any part of his body for prolonged periods.

After Grandpa Hiroshi's funeral, I was worried about how Grandma was coping on her own. I'd learned in medical school that when an elderly person passes away, their spouse often dies within a year or so. Loneliness and heartbreak might be emotions but they affect people physically too, and none is better demonstrated than with this phenomenon. Fourth year was a dedicated research year at uni, and I had a short break before commencing my project so I decided to visit Grandma.

When I rang Grandma's doorbell I could hear the creak of her standing up from her wooden chair and the shuffling of her slippers on the floorboards. 'Coming!' she sang out. She opened the door with a smile so wide her eyes disappeared into her big apple cheeks. She gave me the softest bear hug. I breathed in her cardigan, which smelled like fresh soap and flowers, relieved to see her looking well. I deposited my suitcase in the guest room and came to sit down with her in front of the television. The sumo championships were on.

'I guess you're old enough for this now,' Grandma said as she passed me a dark-blue can of Suntory Rich Malt. I was twenty, the legal age in Japan. Was I really drinking beer and watching sport with my grandma? It felt weird but cool.

After her being with my grandfather for nearly sixty years I could only imagine how lonely she was feeling, but Grandma was trying her best to keep herself occupied. Her father was a painter and her mother had played the organ in a church, so creativity was in my grandmother's genes. I looked over at the kitchen table and noticed that the teapot was wearing a new jacket Grandma had crocheted. Next to the teapot was a sketchbook and some charcoal pencils.

Grandma asked how medical school was. I told her about the very first open-heart surgery I'd watched just a few months before. I'd stood behind the curtains with the anaesthetist, who gave me an Attenborough-style commentary of the surgeon in his natural habitat. It was incredible how the heart was stopped during the operation, and revived at the end. I couldn't believe that in front of me was an open chest with a real-life heart sitting in it.

'Oh Grandma, it was amazing!' I squealed. 'I want to be a surgeon too!'

On this visit I started giving Grandma pedicures. She was getting stiff in her old age and found it difficult to reach her toenails with the clippers. I went to the shops and picked out a bright red nail polish. Grandma wiggled her toes.

'How fun! My toes are dancing!' she said with a gentle giggle.

'They look great, Grandma!'

'I look like a Pan Pan girl!'

'A Pan Pan girl?' I asked.

'During the war, the American soldiers would bring Pan Pan girls red lipstick and nail polish from America,' she explained.

Grandma put on her open-toe sandals to show off her

fresh red coat as we kept chatting during a walk in the neighbouring park.

'Look at the petals on these,' she said, pointing to a white flower with a perfectly symmetrical arrangement.

'What's this one called, Grandma?'

'These are Japanese camellias. They symbolise the bond between mother and child,' she explained, as I gave her hand a tight squeeze.

Back in Sydney, Eriko had just started the second year of her arts/law degree at the University of Sydney and Mariko was in Year 11. Unlike our father, Eriko was engrossed in law and intent on becoming a solicitor after graduation. I too was well and truly immersed in my studies. Nothing could distract me from them. I still kept in touch with Lola but other than her my friends and social life had dissipated because we had been divided into small groups and sent to different hospitals all over Sydney for our placements. Some students were also rotated out to rural hospitals in Wagga Wagga, Port Macquarie, Albury or Coffs Harbour.

Pub crawls and trivia nights were replaced with study groups in the library. Now that we were in fourth year, we were more focused on exams. I continued to enjoy all of my terms. I liked them from an intellectual point of view, but how I felt about surgery was visceral. I loved the adrenaline rush during a fast-paced trauma surgery, the sights and sounds in the operating theatre, and the mechanics of using my hands.

My friend Belinda also had her heart set on surgery. She was really smart, and excelling on the course. She wasn't sure what she wanted to specialise in, but she was spending a lot of time with the General Surgery team. There was gossip that she was favoured by one of its professors, that he was teaching her extra techniques and giving her some private tuition. All the students on my course were thirsty to succeed and be the best. Hearing this talk, it was hard not to feel jealous. The doctors, especially surgeons, were incredibly busy, so often they'd cancel our tutorials, which meant that our ability to learn from them was curtailed. We craved any extra learning we could get but, like the rest of us, Belinda was competitive and it wasn't as if she was going to start sharing her notes from her lessons with this professor. It's easy for the rest of us to say, 'Of course we'd share our notes.' But would we? I might not have been happy to admit it to myself then, but I don't think I would have. And Belinda wasn't exactly in a hurry, either, to ask this professor if he'd take the rest of us for a tutorial.

Some of the students started to gossip about Belinda. It was horrible stuff; about favours she might be giving professors. I hated it. It was as though we were all being pushed by a pernicious envy that was driven by the environment we were in: get ahead, at any cost, and bring down anyone who's getting further ahead. It seemed to get worse as we were entering the second half of medical school; the serious, pointy end. It was always the girls who copped it, too, I noticed. If a male student was liked by a consultant it was because he was an outstanding student. It was never to do with his looks or his behaviour. But somehow if a girl were in the same situation people would make snide remarks. They'd say it was only because she was hot, or, worse, that she was performing sexual favours. All that stuff made my skin crawl, and could make the uni and hospital environment uncomfortable places. The sad thing was, I got used to it. Instead of fighting it, I accepted it because I knew it wouldn't change. I just made a mental note to always wear pants or skirts well below the knee. I wasn't going to let anyone talk about me the way they spoke about Belinda. I was determined to show people that I was succeeding because of my brains and eliminate all other possible factors.

I let my results speak for themselves. Just prior to starting my research project, I found out that I had placed in the top three of my year group in the anatomy exams. Dr Norman selected me and the two others to be demonstrators in the lab, which would mean we'd get to teach anatomy practicals to the first- and second-year medical students. For the first time since starting university, I felt like I'd finally distinguished myself. I think Akuto-san would have been proud of me, and we would've celebrated with a chocolate parfait. When I got home I told my parents, and they congratulated me in their reserved, Japanese manner.

Research hours were flexible, which allowed me to teach a few hours a week. My research area was chronic fatigue syndrome. Since my experience with it, I had determined I would show that there was science to support this phenomenon. My fatigue was definitely real but I wanted my peers to know it, especially Neil. Fern Walker happened to be doing some interesting research with a professor of infectious diseases on chronic fatigue syndrome, which was serendipitous. After my short interaction with her last year, I knew she'd be a supportive supervisor.

The hypothesis Fern and I wanted to prove was that people who suffered from infections such as glandular fever experience changes in their autonomic nervous system, which mediates the sensation of fatigue. I tested the nervous systems of various patients and healthy volunteers.

Fourth year was not what I was expecting. It quickly became obvious to me that I wasn't really suited to research. I much preferred the hustle and bustle of the hospital. I liked being busy and stimulated by the dynamic environment on the wards and operating theatres. Research was a little too slow. It takes time, and I'd always been impatient.

Now that I wasn't spending long hours in rotations at hospitals, I had more spare time, and I decided to fill it with some casual work and volunteering. I signed up to be an aged care volunteer at a nearby hospital. There were elderly patients who were lonely on the wards. Maybe some of them were recently widowed, or didn't have family around, like Grandma. As volunteers we would sit down with them for a chat, and offer help such as moisturising their hands. Many of the elderly patients had dry, neglected skin so we brought bottles of moisturiser with us on our visits.

When I wasn't volunteering, I tutored anatomy at the university. I loved teaching as much as surgery, maybe more. Whether it was debating or Med Show, I thought of myself as an entertainer, and Myers-Briggs confirmed this to be true. Teaching felt a bit like entertaining. I wanted my classes to be fun. I wanted my younger peers to find anatomy as interesting as I did.

The anatomy laboratory was in Room 101, but it was no torture chamber. It was my stage. As I walked into my teaching cubicle, I would pull back the curtains with a flourish and stride in. I felt like this was a safe bubble, in which no one was going to take me down or hate me for knowing too much. The opposite was the case – the students wanted to know more, and I revelled in sharing my knowledge.

The lively engagement of my students encouraged me to want to shine. I took great efforts to prepare for each class, looking back at my notes from the first few years of medical school and reflecting on what I liked about my own teachers. I decided that my favourite teachers were the ones who had the best diagrams, so I practised my drawing every day. I would always get to Room 101 early to draw my diagrams on the blackboard. I liked how the pastel chalks crumbled into a soft powder as I pressed them into the board. Salmon pink arteries and baby blue veins. This was the best of both worlds, where both sides of my brain could harmonise. I think this is why I loved anatomy so much – because I got to study form and shapes.

Teaching helped the year go by quicker. The research was also going well, even if it wasn't my favourite form of learning. When Fern and I did the final data analysis towards the end of the year, we were able to support our hypothesis. At least I knew for sure that what I'd felt was real and there was science to back it up; my findings proved to be a psychological win for me. At the presentations to our peers, I saw Neil in the audience. Even though we'd never said anything to each other about what had happened between us in that second year, I suddenly felt as though I was presenting my research to him alone. *See, Neil? I wasn't faking it. Fatigue is a real thing.*

My experience in second year, and this subsequent study, stirred up some serious questions in me. For one thing I realised how cynical medical people, who are supposed to be the epitome of compassion, can be. I wondered how my peers would treat a patient who presented to them with chronic fatigue. Would they be sceptical, or would they believe the symptoms the patients reported? And I asked myself how I would cope in the future if I became sick. I told myself then that I would never allow myself to get sick if I could help it. The fact this wasn't necessarily realistic didn't occur to me at the time – I simply determined that I wouldn't allow my body to fail me again.

I wanted to publish my research, for two reasons. One, because I believed in it. And two, because everyone told me that you need publications on your CV to succeed. So I kept in touch with Fern and started writing an article on chronic fatigue syndrome for a medical journal. Fern had a few ideas in mind for which journals we could submit my article to. Collecting data during the year had been laborious. Writing was a sweet way to tie everything together, and the thought of seeing my work published was exciting.

7

Knife before life

2009, Sydney

I was twenty-one years old, and as I embarked on my last two years of medical school it seemed a new world. In January Barack Obama was inaugurated as president of the United States. I had hoped he would get elected, all the time wondering if we'd ever see a black man at the helm. Whenever I thought about 'Yes, We Can!' I thought of Bob the Builder first, and then Obama, but nevertheless his campaign had done something to me. I got a lump in my throat every time I thought about it. He was now the most powerful person in the world. You don't need to be a white man to succeed. This was the message I felt the most.

On my first day of fifth year, I stepped into the lift at my new hospital and I felt its buzz as it ascended to the neurosurgical ward. I was buzzing too. I was excited to finally be based at the hospital after a year of sitting in a research office, and of course that I was doing a surgical term. I met my registrars, Janine and

Sam, and Edmund from England, who was doing a fellowship having just passed his final exams as a registrar. The three of them were nice, they always took me out to lunch and made me feel part of the team. Jan in particular spent a lot of time with me. She seemed to care that I was enjoying my term and getting as much learning out of it as possible. As well as teaching me about neurosurgery, she gave me some general advice to help me become a good intern, too – tips such as ensuring I made referrals to other specialties before 10 am. 'Registrars are busy so the earlier you refer the better, then they can fit the referral into their day,' she told me.

The consultants were an interesting and entertaining bunch. They all had a phrase: 'knife before wife'. Since I didn't have a wife, I adapted it to create my own motto for surgery: 'knife before life'. Soon I gained a reputation among my fellow students for being like the surgery-crazy Cristina Yang from *Grey's Anatomy*.

One Friday, one of the orthopaedic registrars started talking to me. 'Why are you here on a Friday? The other students are probably all at the beach.'

'Why wouldn't I be here? It's just another normal weekday.'

'Look at how nice it is outside, though. Is it because you're an international student? Need to get bang for your buck, do ya?'

Ugh, I regretted that he knew that information. I wished that I had a tag on my shirt that read: 'International student, but will be staying in Australia to work in the public system, so please teach me!' The orthopaedic registrar was Asian himself, but he'd grown up in Australia. Somehow that made him superior to me. I hated this feeling. Would I always be made to feel 'international'? I desperately wanted to be the same as everyone else. I mean, I sounded like a local, so that conferred a slight advantage over other international students who were heavily accented, but apparently I still wasn't an Aussie.

The next week I asked Edmund to show me how to do hand ties, and a nurse for some 3-0 Vicryl ties to practise with. I opened the packet of purple threads for my impromptu lesson. Edmund was extremely patient with me. He watched carefully as I tied each knot, and took me through the technique step by step until I got it perfectly. I was walking on cloud nine after that session. I loved learning new surgical skills. It made me feel as though I was inching closer to my dreams.

'Jan!' I yelled out as I caught up with her for lunch. 'Edmund taught me hand ties!'

'Hey, matey! That's great,' she said, patting me on the shoulder.

Janine was down to earth. The patients liked that she was casual with them. She called them 'mate' and talked to them as though they were swigging beers at the pub. Sam said she needed to be more refined. She had applied for the neurosurgery training program and would be sitting interviews in a few months.

'You have to look a certain way,' Jan explained. 'All the chicks have their hair in French chignons and wear pearls.'

I took mental notes. Chignon. Pearls. Her literal pearls of wisdom. It would still be several years before I'd have to apply for the plastic surgery training program, but I stored that piece of advice in the back of my head, where I stored all the other tips Jan had shared. I still had to finish medical school and do my internship and residency before even thinking about specialty programs. It still seemed far away before I'd need to practise doing my hair in a chignon.

At home I practised hand ties for hours – on any handle I could find in our house. Soon they were all covered with purple braids and Yoshiko, who was usually a clean freak, didn't make me remove them. I could tell she was smiling as she watched me hone my skills. My parents never got in the way of me doing anything that related to my aspirations of becoming a surgeon. Those purple braids were a part of our interior décor until we moved out of that house.

My obsession with surgery grew stronger during that term. I took every opportunity to go to the operating theatre and attend surgical clinics. I was lucky to have a colorectal surgeon, Dr Stein, as my clinical tutor for my final two years. He could see that I was keen and he let me follow him around like his shadow everywhere he went. He was a brilliant teacher and had a way of emphasising important things so that we wouldn't forget them. For example, he simplified hernias for us. The anatomy of hernias in the groin is quite complicated, but he summarised it simply: 'If the lump is below the inguinal ligament, it's a femoral hernia. If it's not, it's inguinal.'

One afternoon I went to one of his operating lists. I hovered near his shoulder to try to see what he was doing. He suddenly stopped. 'Yumiko! It might be more important for *me* to see since I'm the one doing the operation,' he laughed.

'Oops, sorry,' I replied and retreated. I hadn't noticed that my eager, bobbing head was blocking his view.

'You're ready to start operating, aren't you?' he said. 'I can just feel you wanting to take over this one.'

One Dr Stein-ism that I never forgot was a lesson about how he ended up in proctology – the marvellous sub-specialty of bums. His advice was that in order to be successful you should pick something that no one else wanted to do and be really good at it, so that you became the expert in it. And for sure, if anyone were to suffer from haemorrhoids or anal fissures, I couldn't think of anyone else I'd refer them to. I did think to myself, though, why can't I choose something popular like plastic surgery and still become the best at it?

Some days, I followed Dr Stein's registrar Ingrid around. I noticed her blonde hair was in a perfect chignon every day, and her earlobes were adorned with large pearls. My god, Jan was not joking! Ingrid wore rimless glasses and her eyes were always lined with a sharp streak of liquid eyeliner. She looked so chic and composed, but she always seemed to be angry, especially with the radiology department.

'What's the fucking delay?' she'd yell down the phone. 'We needed the fucking CT scan this morning. This guy needs to go to surgery.'

One day I asked her why she got so cross at radiology. 'There's no room for wallflowers in surgery,' she said. 'Especially if you're a girl.'

I pondered that for a moment, and it kept me thinking. Did we really need to behave like that? I knew that it was harder to be a female in surgery, but was I going to have to start shouting at people to fit in? I didn't want to be like that. Surely there was a way of being assertive without being rude? I wondered whether Ingrid had always had an angry streak, or whether it was working in Surgery that made her behave like that.

*

Around this time, Fern was promoted from senior lecturer to associate professor. I went to see her to congratulate her. She was pleased but frustrated. 'Took bloody forever,' she explained. 'Younger men have come through and been given promotions much quicker than me. A few of my colleagues really had to push hard for me to get this.'

I sat there, nodding, not sure how to respond. I had no idea how academic promotions worked, or how hard it had been for her. Fern's gold glasses glistened in the afternoon sun streaming through her window. Today she had pink roses in her hair and a frilly red dress.

'You do all this research and teaching, but it's hard to get any recognition,' she said. 'The university doesn't take me seriously.'

I hoped Fern's flowery outfits and out-there personality had nothing to do with that. I realised that when I thought of what the world considered 'professorial', it was plaid jackets with elbow patches, and bow ties.

'Anyway,' she said. 'I have some good news. Our paper has been accepted!'

My eyes lit up like LED lights. Fern and I celebrated with biscuits and tea. I left her office feeling on top of the world.

8

Konjo

2010, Sydney

I had less than half a year left until medical school graduation.
I was raring to go, like a shiny ball in a pinball machine, though
amid my cohort's excitement at the idea of finishing and passing
the course, I was a little concerned about internship positions
for the following year. There was a lot at stake. Completing an internship was absolutely crucial. Without a position,
I wouldn't be registered by the Medical Board to practise as
a doctor, essentially making my medical degree defunct. The
federal government had over-reacted to the doctor shortage
and created more medical school spots without increasing
the number of postgraduate training positions. The facepalm
situation was called the 'medical student tsunami' and my
intake of 2005 was the start of it. In New South Wales, appli-
cants were prioritised according to tiers. The top tier was for
local students who had attended a New South Wales medical
school. The second was for local students who'd completed

Year 12 in the state, but went to an interstate medical school, and so on. As an international student, I was at the bottom of the barrel. I was told that international students would not be guaranteed any jobs when first-round offers were announced. My competence didn't matter because internship positions were decided using a utilitarian ballot system.

I decided to apply for hospitals in Melbourne, which used a merit-based system. I had Dr Stein as a referee, and I thought my CV was strong. I was also buoyed by a recent nomination for a prize. The Department of Anatomy had nominated me for a Vice Chancellor's Award for Teaching Excellence. As a student tutor, I never would have thought I'd even be considered for this accolade. In fact, I didn't know such awards existed at the university. Every little thing helped when competition for internships was fierce. After looking at all the different hospitals in Melbourne, my heart was set on one of the big networks, which had an excellent reputation for a wide range of specialties and, importantly, a Plastic Surgery unit. I sent the hospital my CV and reference reports and kept my fingers crossed that I'd be called for interviews.

In May I was offered one. I didn't know what kind of questions I'd be asked, but I brought a fire in me. That's all twenty-two-year-old me had – what the Japanese call *konjo*. It means to approach everything with guts, drawing inspiration from the samurai spirit. It's a source of criticism for Japanese people in areas like sport. Instead of being guided by science and evidence, courage, effort and spirit were favoured. True enough, I didn't know how the interview was structured, nor how to prepare for it, but I did know that I would be able to convey my passion and dedication to Medicine.

*

My next term in Sydney was in Emergency. Each of us was allocated to a registrar – mine was a senior registrar called Kieran. We were to follow our registrar for all his or her shifts, including night shifts. Most of the term consisted of drunks punching each other, coming in as pairs, one with a broken jaw and the other with a broken hand from punching that jaw. Witnessing the work and patient behaviour in Emergency made me appreciate nurses and how much they had to put up with. Sometimes people who came in would get the alcohol runs so they'd literally be shitting everywhere while being shit-faced, flooding the ED floor with a river of shit.

As the senior registrar, Kieran was often busy on night shifts because he was in charge and staffing was scarce, unlike day shifts when there were consultants in charge and more doctors to share the workload. I observed and made myself useful where possible. There was a lot of unpredictability. Occasionally it was so quiet that you could hear the hum of a computer; other times paramedics would rush in with patients on stretchers, one after the other. There was one night when a cardiac transplant was taking place, so I asked for Kieran's permission to go and watch it. I went upstairs to the operating theatres, where the chill of the air conditioning blasting through the empty space and the anticipation of the precious heart arriving from its donor created a frozen stillness. As soon as the heart was carried into the operating theatre in its courier bag, sound and movement returned. Moments like this made me feel like surgery was such an incredible gift to be able to give someone. These two small size-six hands of mine could one day perform operations that would make a difference to someone's life.

I walked back down to the ED to see chaos in the resuscitation bay. A middle-aged woman was struggling to breathe. She was sitting bolt upright with an oxygen mask to her face, and she looked weary as each breath became more and more laboured. She was going to need an emergency tracheostomy so they were waiting for the ear, nose and throat registrar, Chris, to come in. When he arrived, I ran after him and asked if I could follow him up to theatres as I'd never seen a tracheostomy before. 'You can do it, if you like,' he said. My eyes lit up like neon dreams. I got approval from Kieran, so I sprinted to the operating theatre for the second time that night, the excitement pulsing through my veins.

Chris had a calm demeanour. Even though this was an emergency surgery, which normally meant medical students were shoved out of the way, he'd invited me right into the centre of the action. Some doctors like to teach, others don't. Lucky for me Chris was the former, and he instructed me while I performed my first tracheostomy. The scrub nurse handed me a scalpel. I looked at Chris, who nodded with encouragement. I made a careful cut across the base of the woman's neck. I felt calm and my hands were steady. I'd studied the anatomy of the neck; I'd watched videos and live surgeries. I'd been preparing for a moment like this for years. I used some blunt scissors to dissect down to the trachea. Wow, this is surgery. A plastic tube was placed into the trachea and now all that was left was to secure the tube to the skin.

'Can you hand tie?' asked Chris. Oh, can I ever!

'Yup,' I replied, trying to be cool about it, but inside I was squealing, relishing my chance to finally shine. I tied the first suture, making sure each knot was squared perfectly.

'Very good. Can you tie with your left hand?' Yes! Yes! I was jumping up and down on the inside. The hours I'd spent tying 3-0 Vicryl ties around my parents' house were coming to fruition. I'd tied with my right hand, then my left, with my eyes closed, and then with my hands behind my back. Here was my chance to do it in real life. I tied the second knot with my left hand, nearly as quickly as I had done with my right.

'Now you're just showing off!' said Chris with a hint of a smile under his mask. Before I knew it the case was over and I had performed my first tracheostomy under supervision. I thanked Chris profusely.

I met Chris later again in his career when he became a consultant. He couldn't remember me but I thanked him again for that opportunity. To him it was just a little gesture, but for me it was the highlight of my entire term.

After the operation, I ran back downstairs to finish the night shift. Things had quietened down in the Emergency Department.

'How was it?' Kieran asked.

'Oh, it was great! Chris let me do the tracheostomy!' I gushed, trying not to sound too excited, because I didn't want Kieran to think that I was more interested in attending surgeries than learning from the ED, but I think he already knew that.

It was a chilly day in July when the internship offers arrived. Not unexpectedly, I did not get a job in New South Wales. After six long years of studying and learning in the hospital environment, NSW Health hadn't given me a position. Even though it wasn't a surprise, I still felt really frustrated, and a bit worried. My feeling of disenfranchisement was, however,

short-lived. I opened my emails and ... 'MAMA! PAPA!'
I screamed as I ran down the corridor to the living room
where they were watching rugby on the television. I stood in
front of them, jumping, arms flailing uncontrollably. 'I got the
Melbourne internship! I got it!' I kept screaming for another
ten minutes until I was winded. They couldn't not let me go
unless they wanted me to be unemployed. In a rare display of
affection, both of my parents hugged me. I could tell that they
were happy and proud. I was going to Victoria!

My final term before graduation was Colorectal Surgery. It was
great to get Dr Stein as a teacher again. Mentors were hard
enough to come by, so having one like Dr Stein to work with
every day was amazing. We started each morning at 7 so we
could see all of the inpatients. One night I stayed until late
to watch an abdominoperineal resection, which involves the
removal of cancer in the lower rectum. After this had been
done, I was given the tricky job of suturing the perineum
back together. But I was keen to do more. During the next
part of the surgery the end of the colon is brought outside
the body through the skin of the abdomen to create what's
called the stoma. It was a bit cheeky of me, but when the
surgeon was doing this, I asked if I could put a stitch in. 'Okay,
but just a couple,' he said. I thanked him and carefully threaded
the prolene stitch through the bowel and sutured it to the skin.

I left the operating theatre that night feeling overjoyed. The
registrar Ingrid told me not to come in the next morning for
ward rounds because I had stayed back, but I still came, of
course.

Over the two years, Dr Stein had got to know me well. He knew how fervently I wanted to pursue surgery and he'd always been supportive of that. At this stage I wasn't confident about telling anyone, including him, that I wanted to do Plastics, since I hadn't done a term in it as a doctor yet, but I knew that when I was ready to tell him he'd be happy for me. We went out for a farewell drink and I got tipsy on one mojito, which he found amusing. After a few sips, my face had turned pink. It's a defect in the alcohol dehydrogenase enzyme. The Oriental flush.

'Dr Stein, I'm going to be a surgeon,' I said in my happy mojito haze.

'Well, of course you are! You didn't do all that hard work here not to become a surgeon, did you?' he asked.

'No,' I replied, smiling through my white rum blush. I sculled the rest of my mojito and headed home. I knew that Dr Stein would be a mentor for life.

The class of 2010 gathered in mid-December for our graduation. It was uncommon for me to celebrate my academic achievements with my parents, but on this occasion I felt I'd earned it: I was graduating with honours. I had made it to the end of medical school, and I allowed myself to fully absorb this moment. My sisters were proud of me, and I was proud of them: Eriko was now in her penultimate year of her law degree, and Mariko had just finished high school. I looked around the auditorium, which was humming with nostalgia. For six years I had walked in and out of this auditorium for lectures, and even got to see what it was like back stage for the Med

Shows I had performed in. Today it was full of proud parents, grandparents, siblings, spouses, and of course our teachers. There was still that competitive commotion over who'd been awarded honours and who hadn't, but we were all happy for each other as we sat in our chairs waiting for our moment in the sun.

After collecting our hard-earned degrees, we walked outside for the obligatory mortarboard-tossing photos. My elation was cut short and my smile faded as I saw Prof Dubia out of the corner of my eye. I tried to manoeuvre myself away, but he snaked his way around the students between us.

'Yumiko,' he called out. I shuddered, as though I was hearing the creepy 'Greensleeves' tune from an ice-cream truck. 'Congratulations,' he said, holding out his wrinkled hand. I wanted to spit on it. If it weren't for the other students surrounding us, I would have.

'Thank you, Professor Dubia,' I said in a measured voice, as I stared at him with empty eyes. His sleazy gaze was magnified behind his thick bifocal lenses. How dare he show up at my graduation ceremony. Who else did he hope to see? Who else had he wanted to touch? I was really disappointed to see that he was still an appointed professor at the university, but at least I was leaving Sydney for my internship. No one could take away from my graduation day. I'd worked hard, and now I was going to be a doctor.

PART 2

Intern

9

I'm sorry to bother you

2011, Victoria

Yumiko. Twenty-three. Doctor. It was finally happening. I looked down at my new iPhone 4 as 'Mum' appeared on its glossy black screen. My parents were calling to say they were just around the corner from my new share house. They had driven down to Melbourne from Sydney to help me move. Yoshiko made sure my pantry was well stocked: light and dark soy sauce, rice cooking wine, mirin, and everything else a good Japanese girl should have in her kitchen. After ensuring each bottle was placed neatly, she looked at me with sadness in her eyes, a forced smile on her face. 'Work hard, Yumiko.' It felt bittersweet, a bit like mirin. Becoming a doctor was my dream come true, but this was the first time I'd ever lived in a different house from my family, let alone a different city.

My new housemates were Sasha, who was starting internship at the same hospital as me, and Rory, an engineer I knew through a friend.

The next morning I timed my commute, and watched as a helicopter landed on the roof above the Emergency Department. I imagined the unfolding scenario. A cardiac transplant? A multi-trauma patient from a rural hospital? A patient with severe burns? I couldn't believe I was going to be a part of all this soon.

Although . . . I'd have to wait ten weeks – I had been allocated an Emergency term in rural Victoria as my first rotation. Most interns do at least one rural rotation but I wished it didn't have to be for my first term – I wanted to settle into my new place, explore this new city and get to know the other interns I'd be working alongside.

A few weeks before, I'd been sent a perfunctory email with things I needed to know for my first rotation, such as the address of the hospital and the intern house where I'd be living for the next ten weeks. Other than that, I was expecting to turn up and figure everything out when I got there.

I had to google the town in Victoria to find out where I was heading – a small place a few hours from Melbourne. At the internship orientation, I found my peers who'd be with me. There was Lily from Adelaide; John from Perth; Aaron, who went to Melbourne University; and Martha from Monash University. John was the most outgoing of the bunch, and the youngest. We shared the same birthday but he was a year younger than me. His medical degree had been five years, while mine was six because of the compulsory research year we had to do. The competitive part of me was a bit jealous that he might become a specialist at a younger age than me. At twenty-three, I was still considered relatively young to be a doctor, but I couldn't help myself – I always felt like I was competing. There tends to be admiration for the youngest person to achieve X or Y, like they're some sort of genius or prodigy. I asked John what he wanted to do in the future. He said gastroenterology. Phew.

I started talking to a couple of Asian girls. It's possible that was a subconscious choice since we were the striking minority: when I looked around the room I could count on my hands the number of non-white people. It was very different from medical school, which had a majority Asian population. It made me think of the bamboo ceiling. Was this the start of it? The higher we climb, the fewer opportunities there might be. Medicine valued qualities such as leadership, which Asians traditionally do worse in. There's this trope of the submissive, timid Asian who doesn't aspire to lead. This docility myth hurts Asian women even more.

Fei had a strong Singaporean accent that I recognised straightaway. I told her I'd grown up in Singapore and we bonded about how much we loved the place. Similarly, Asmah had a distinct Malaysian accent. The three of us continued to chat over the lunchbreak.

While I was helping myself to some sandwiches, an intern who hadn't introduced himself yet walked up to me. 'Do you have Ehlers-Danlos syndrome?' he asked. Mate, I don't even know your name and you're already diagnosing me with a syndrome? Either his university hadn't taught their students bedside manners, or this guy had no social skills. He continued, 'I noticed you have a scar on your left arm. That's the typical place where children get pilomatrixomas. Did you have a pilomatrixoma? I want to be a rheumatologist, you see.'

He was indeed correct. I'd had a small skin tumour removed from that spot. I nodded politely and excused myself to say hello to some of the other interns. Suffice to say, none of them mentioned skin tumours.

The atmosphere in those first days in Melbourne as all the interns got to know each other was sociable and upbeat. I was excited to make new friends and decided to hold an interns' party in our shared house. Rory owned an impressive set of speakers so he was our resident DJ. I laughed and danced all night and did the worm a few times – my one and only party trick. I took lots of photos with my fellow interns on my camera. 'Yeah, the interns!' I screamed as we all raised our plastic cups. I wished I wasn't leaving Melbourne immediately so that I could spend more time with new friends like Fei and Asmah. Some interns were being seconded to other hospitals, but most were starting at our base.

I didn't have my driver's licence so John had offered me a lift to the rural posting – we'd be doing Emergency together as our first rotation. He played some nineties R&B in the car. We sang and laughed for the entire journey.

The town we were in had one main street with a Thai restaurant, a supermarket and some shops scattered here and there. We arrived at the intern house, which we would call home for the next ten weeks. Martha was doing a GP term so she was set up in a different house. John and I would be sharing the house with Lily, who was allocated to Medicine, and Aaron, who was doing Surgery. It was a shabby old house, but at least we each got our own rooms. I was lucky enough to get my own shower, in fact, but the other three had to share a bathroom. I'm not sure how I lucked out with that one – perhaps because I would be doing irregular hours as an ED intern, alternating between day and evening shifts, so it was better for me to get my own bathroom and not to bother the others when I got home late at night.

Day one. In the ED John and I were greeted by the two consultants, Adrian and Darren, who gave us a tour of the department and allocated us our first patients. My first real patient! My own patient! He was a young man who had stepped onto some shattered glass, and my job was to pick the glass out of his foot. Ground-breaking medicine, I know. My second patient had a tick on his back. Adrian gave me a few tips on how to get it off with the side of some scissor blades. Success! I proudly put the tick into a little yellow urine jar and showed the patient the creature that had been stuck to him.

When I got back to the intern house that afternoon, I wrote about my first day in my journal. Eriko had given me a 365-day diary for Christmas, and I was determined to fill every day with my internship chronicles. I decided that I would write all of my entries with my non-dominant left hand. I remember Dr Stein insisting I learn to do with my left hand everything I could do with my right. 'Sometimes your right hand will be deep in a patient's abdominal cavity retracting some bowel, so you need to be able to do things like use scissors with your left hand,' he'd explained. It had certainly paid off with the knot-tying.

The second week was much like the first, filled with mundane ailments. Things were going well until the Thursday. There was a lady with nondescript abdominal symptoms. I didn't quite know what was wrong with her, but I followed the usual principles to try to reach a diagnosis: I took a thorough history and examined her carefully. I ordered a number of basic blood tests and was waiting upon their results when a nurse, Candace, pulled me aside. 'You're not communicating with your patient. All you've done is order some tests and not told her anything.' It was my first criticism as a doctor, and it was hard for me to take. I'd always considered myself a good communicator, so to be pulled up in this particular way stung. It was a jolt of a reminder that I still had a lot to learn, and improvements to make.

On Friday evening a middle-aged man, Malcolm, came in with his wife, Julia. They had been to another smaller hospital in the area earlier that day, where Malcolm was told that he had mild heatstroke before being discharged and advised to keep hydrated and cool. He had ongoing symptoms, though, so the couple was worried and had brought him into this ED. Candace was on the same shift with me again, so I saw it as an opportunity to prove to her that I *could* communicate.

Malcolm had had a headache all day, without any history of trauma. His eyes also felt a bit blurry. The fact that he had re-presented to another hospital was a red flag and I knew that I needed to be very detailed in my assessment. I took great care in checking his cranial nerves, and noticed that there was something wrong with his right eye. I was alarmed that it wasn't moving like his left. As students we learn how to do examinations on each other, and we see abnormal signs in patients who have already been diagnosed, but this was the first time I was the first to pick up an abnormality. *I'm a doctor now. I diagnose people.* I felt the gravity of this as I documented the third cranial nerve palsy. This was no heatstroke. Mindful of

Candace's criticism the day before, I explained my findings to Malcolm and Julia, informing them that a number of things could cause these eye signs, that I'd be calling a senior colleague for help, and arranging for Malcolm to have a CT scan of his head.

I called the medical registrar and proceeded to organise an urgent CT scan. As it was nearly 10 pm, I was nervous and apologetic because I felt bad ringing someone at that time of night. However, the registrar was nice about it and came in straight away as though it was no bother. I also had to call the after-hours radiographer, who'd need to set up the scanning machine. By the time I'd finished writing in Malcolm's medical notes, the registrar had arrived. He assessed Malcolm and confirmed my findings. 'Make sure that CT scan happens ASAP,' he instructed, in a soft but firm voice.

Malcolm's scan was done but there were no radiologists to report on it. I could see a big area of bleeding at the back of his brain. Jan, Sam and Edmund had taught me well during my Neurosurgery term. The registrar advised that I call the Melbourne hospitals as a matter of urgency to transfer Malcolm for neurosurgical care. It was getting late at night and, again, I was a little nervous about calling the on-call registrars in Melbourne. I knew that I had to present the case succinctly.

I explained to Malcolm and Julia that there was blood on Malcolm's brain, which is likely what had caused his headache and visual symptoms, and that he would need more specialised care in the city. Then I called the Melbourne hospital that had this one in its catchment area. I reminded myself of the ISBAR method of communicating with colleagues: *Introduce* yourself and the patient. *Situation*: what is going on. *Background* of the patient's medical history. *Assessment*: what I think the problem is. *Recommendation*: ask what is recommended.

I took a deep breath and called the first hospital switchboard to ask them to put me through to the neurosurgical registrar, my heart pounding louder with every ring. A male voice picked up.

'Hello, I'm so sorry to bother you,' I began as my standard greeting. Sorry. It was the Japanese part of me, I couldn't help it. Others might wonder why Japanese people apologise all the time, but to me it's normal, polite. When we go to our friends' houses, we say, 'Sorry to disturb you,' even though we're the ones invited over. We say, 'Sorry this is so small,' when giving a gift we've spent generously on. The groupthink of Japanese people can be ridiculous. It's an extreme and deranged level of self-lowering to make others feel better, more comfortable, or superior even, to the point where it can turn into a bargaining tool. I say sorry to soften the blow of what I'm about to ask, hoping that it might make the answer a 'yes'.

'I'm Yumiko, I'm an intern. Sorry to call so late,' I apologised again. 'I —'

'We have no beds,' he interjected abruptly before I could even ask. Okay, then . . . I guess I'll have to try another hospital. And so the circuit of phone calls around Melbourne began.

When you go to medical school, you learn about diagnosing and treating diseases. You don't learn about administrative hurdles such as bed availability. That night every major hospital in Melbourne seemed to be bed-blocked. I grew more and more twitchy with each phone call. I thought of what that registrar Ingrid had told me as a final-year medical student: there are no wallflowers in surgery. As such a junior intern, I felt timid, but I knew I needed to get that bed for Malcolm, so I decided I needed to speak a bit more assertively.

My next phone call was to a lovely registrar from Melbourne's St Vincent's, who unfortunately had the same bed situation. 'I'm sorry, we don't have beds, but if you have any problems you can ring me again.' Finally. Someone nice.

I updated Malcolm and Julia on what was happening. I had tried five hospitals and they were all full, so I decided to ring back the registrar from St Vincent's, who accepted care of Malcolm and requested I send through a copy of the images. I was so relieved and grateful for the one sympathetic registrar. I spoke to the nurse in charge about organising an urgent air transfer to Melbourne and went back to Malcolm and Julia to give them another update. At some point during all of this, I thought to myself, *I'm really overdoing it*. But I've since learned that there is no such thing as communicating too much with a patient. Of course, you don't want to overload people with information, especially filled with medical jargon, but keeping patients and family members in the loop reduces anxiety and the long waits wondering what's happening.

When I got home, I grabbed my pen with my left hand and wrote clumsily in my diary my account of the day. It was going to take a while before I could write smoothly with my non-dominant hand. I was glad that Candace had said something to me about communicating better with my patients, because I felt that I had really tried hard to take care of Malcolm. And I think that for an intern I did all right.

10

Do I scrub up all right?

2011, Victoria

What does it mean to be a good doctor? In those early days – but of course all through my med training at uni, too – I would ask myself this, and we would be asked to consider it. In essence, I had come to realise over the last six years that I wanted to be someone in whom a patient could put their whole trust, who made you feel comforted when you felt vulnerable. Importantly, as I was finding out, I had to be able to communicate effectively. However, the next major incident had nothing to do with communication. The patient couldn't communicate because he was dead, and had been for about three days. Having to pronounce someone dead was what I dreaded the most about my intern year. I knew it would be confronting and I was afraid of my emotions. *What if I cry? What if I freak out?* It wasn't something I'd thought about at the start of medical school. It was only in sixth year that we had a tutorial on how to certify death. It was then that I had to really face up to the fact that it was going to be a part of the job.

I was the only doctor in the hospital when the co-ordinator barged into the ED with her very important-looking folder clutched to her bosom.

'Where's the intern?'

'That's me,' I replied.

'Come with me now. The police have brought a body into the morgue and you need to certify him.' It seemed I had no choice in the matter. I was scared, but I knew that I couldn't say no . . . or could I? I had no time to think as she rushed me into a silent corridor. It was early in the morning and there were hardly any staff members in the hospital. The click-clack of her very important shoes echoed dissonantly with the drag of my inexperienced sneakers. My stethoscope hung heavily around my neck, and my little torch was getting sweaty in my palm. I could feel my pulse in my ears and could smell rotting flesh before we turned a tight corner.

'The police think he's been dead for a few days now,' she said in her very important voice. 'He left a note on his car that read "Dead body ahead, contact police".' That crushed my heart. This man, even moments before deciding to kill himself, was thoughtful. He didn't want a civilian to find a dead body. The putridity punched my nose when I walked into the morgue. 'I trust you know how to get back to the Emergency Department,' said the hospital co-ordinator. She walked out leaving a trail of very important perfume, which mingled with the smell of decay.

Two police officers stood on either side of the body. I stared at the dead man in front of me. He was about my age. He had fired a gun through his mouth. His head was swollen and deformed from the gun shot. The exit wound was on the upper right part of his skull, and a nest of maggots was wriggling in it. I had never seen anything like it. It was like a scene from a horror film. I didn't know whether I was shivering because I was cold, or because I was mortified at what my eyes were seeing, what my nose was smelling. My senses were overwhelmed, but I knew what I needed to do.

My mind went into autopilot as I started the process of certifying the death. Pupils, must check the pupils. I held up my torch and one of his eyelids. Some maggots crawled out, and I silently gasped. One of the police officers looked at my torch and smirked. 'I don't think you'll be needing that, love.'

My heart was beating a hundred beats a minute, maybe faster. I felt like I was suffocating in this small morgue. I looked at the papers on the desk. 'Just tell me where I need to sign,' I pleaded. I scribbled my signature on the relevant sections and left swiftly. I knew then that the man's body was an image I would never forget.

The senior doctors started an hour later, and I told Adrian all about the ordeal and how I'd been frogmarched to the morgue by the hospital co-ordinator. I walked to my bike to ride home. Some bastard had stolen the light off my handlebar. I rode home in the dark and that night I dreamed about maggots.

Next morning, I caramelised some pear to eat with my French toast for breakfast and found that the slices of pear looked like maggots swimming in a pond of brown sugar. When I arrived at the hospital, I was told that the medical director of the hospital had asked for a meeting with me. He had heard about my experience and wanted to check that

I was all right. I was. But I was furious at the hospital coordinator – how could she do that to an intern? At least I'd never seen the man alive – I didn't know what he was like, or his family circumstances. That would have made it harder. But I couldn't un-see the decomposing body with its violent wound. The medical director asked if I needed counselling. *Counselling?* Did they think I was a wuss who couldn't handle her first death? I declined. I didn't want them to think I was weak. I was a strong and competent intern; there was no way I was going to say yes. I convinced myself I felt fine.

I wondered if, back in Melbourne, junior staff would've had to do a certification like that. I was pretty sure senior doctors would have to take on the responsibility. So I was relieved to hear the medical director reassure me that the hospital had already created a protocol detailing that if a corpse were to come to the morgue overnight, the certification would be done by a senior doctor at the start of their shift, and not by an intern.

A few weeks later, I caught up with Martha. She and I had bonded immediately over our mutual love of surgery. Most of our internship cohort was interested in physicians' training, so I was happy to have met Martha; I knew we would stick together, and her GP rotation made it easy for us to catch up pretty regularly as her shifts were a standard nine to five each day. Martha was a bit older than the rest of us, having done a PhD in Surgery. Her thesis was on colorectal cancer and her supervisor was an eminent professor of general surgery. She had also published an impressive list of articles in well-known journals. So she was already a cut above the rest of us.

That day, a patient had asked me whether I was old enough to be a doctor. I bet no one had asked John that, even though he was younger than me. I wondered how long it would be before I would stop having to prove myself to others. It was hard enough being at the bottom of the pecking order, without having to worry about whether patients thought I was qualified to treat them. Martha had other concerns.

'GP is way too slow for me,' she said. 'The best part is getting to watch surgeries.'

'You mean the procedures they do in the clinic?' I asked.

'No, at the hospital. The rural GPs do Anaesthetics as well,' she explained. 'So I followed my GP to the hospital to watch him do the anaesthesia for one of the operating lists.'

'Oh, I'm jealous! That's so cool. I miss seeing surgeries.'

'I can't wait for my Surgery term,' said Martha.

Nor could I. ED here probably wasn't as slow as Martha's experience in GP, but it lacked the excitement I got from surgery. I was holding out for that rotation, which was at the end of the year. Mine was in Upper Gastrointestinal Surgery, one of the sub-specialties of General Surgery, along with Breast and Endocrine, which Martha was allocated, and Colorectal.

Martha was a shoo-in for the General Surgery training program. We spoke about what we needed to do to get onto the Program – she'd be applying for General Surgery, and I wanted to apply for Plastics. There was a list of courses that would get us points. Over coffee one day Martha took out her laptop and we scrolled through the various courses. There was one on research and surgical literature, one on the emergency management of severe trauma, one on looking after sick surgical patients, and one on surgical skills. Three thousand dollars each. Ouch. People often get asked what they'll spend their first pay cheque on. My answer was surgical courses.

Lily from Adelaide was the other girl I got to know. She was interested in Anaesthesia. Soon after we arrived, Lily and I decided to build a running routine. For our first run around a track near the intern house, I was trailing behind her, gasping for air, while Lily was able to talk and run at the same time. I'd perhaps enjoyed myself a little too much after the end of medical school and was rather unfit, but from then on I went running most days of the week, and soon I was able to keep up with Lily over the 3 kilometres of the track, and even hold a conversation with her. John suggested we do the Run for Kids when we were all back in Melbourne – a 14-kilometre fun run. I'd never run any further than 5 kilometres, but I was always up for a challenge and it felt great to be exercising again so I signed up and kept on training.

On 11 March 2011 one of the worst earthquakes the world had ever recorded hit Tohoku, in the north-east of Japan. The 9.0 magnitude triggered a devastating tsunami, which killed more than 15,000 people, and damaged the Fukushima Nuclear Power Plant. It was the second worst nuclear disaster after Chernobyl. I called my grandmother Naoko straight away. She was well away from the epicentre, but I needed to know that she was okay. With Japan sitting on such a precarious arrangement of tectonic plates, Grandma had lived through many an earthquake. During this one she had felt the ground move and lost electricity for about an hour, but she was thankfully fine. I was speechless as I watched the footage on the television after the phone call. I had never seen such black water before. It didn't seem real as the charcoal-coloured waves swept over towns, lifting homes and cars off the ground.

The heartbreaking pictures from Japan put me in a solemn mood that weekend, but with just a week left of the term I had a nice surprise waiting for me on the Monday morning. The Emergency Department had received a thank-you card from Malcolm and Julia. Malcolm was now in rehab and recovering well from his brain bleed. It was such wonderful news. Adrian was brimming with pride. 'We hardly ever get cards in Emergency departments, because patients don't spend long enough with us to really appreciate what we do,' he said. My first card as a doctor. My eyes were shiny black beads glistening in the cold fluorescent lights of the Emergency Department. I wrote all about it in my diary. I couldn't write fast enough with my left hand, and I punctured the page with all the exclamation points!

I finished the term with full marks in my end-of-term assessment, to the envy of the other interns. 'How did you manage that?' Aaron asked. He didn't think there was any way an intern could be distinguished from others so early in the year. I was delighted – it was a shot of confidence and made me determined to keep getting excellent marks and stand out from the crowd, as I'd tried to all my life.

I finished my shift at 4 pm that day so I decided to go for one last run. I ran five laps of the track. Fifteen kilometres. It was hard and I was slow, but 15 kilometres is 15 kilometres. I was on a high. Thinking about that first short, difficult run with Lily, I was so pleased with my final effort.

That night we went to the local nightclub with Mark, one of the surgical registrars. The dancefloor was dirty and sticky with spilled drinks. There was UV lighting. We danced to Top 40 music and had some drinks. I wore a short grey dress and, unfortunately, white underpants. Inebriated Yumiko decided to do the worm on the disgusting floor, her hands feeling the tackiness of the lino, and her dress collecting black smudges from the soles of strangers' shoes. I knew I was flashing the crowd, which was half-cheering for my worm and half-cheering for my glow-in-the-dark underpants. I guess I was the glow-worm that night. Mark and I danced for a long time, and I could see John grinning and raising his eyebrows cheekily. I shook my head at John. Mark wasn't my type.

The next morning, Martha came over to the intern house to hang out in my room before we all had to leave. We made plans to catch up again in Melbourne. Martha was a bikram yoga regular at a popular studio in Fitzroy. She loved it and was keen to introduce me to it. I was so glad to have made a Melbourne friend who could show me things in my new city.

Later, Mark came to say goodbye to us. As I was stuffing my suitcase with the last of my cotton socks, I heard John say, 'She normally dresses like a guy, but she scrubs up all right, eh?'

'Yeah, man. When she puts in the effort, she's not bad,' Mark replied.

'Did your night finish off with a ... bang?' asked John suggestively.

'Not as big a bang as I would've liked,' said Mark.

Martha and I looked at each other and rolled our eyes. Why did men think it was cool to talk about 'banging' women?

'John's an idiot,' she said.

'Yup,' I agreed. 'Why would I dress up for work anyway? ED's gross. And Mark's gross. They're both gross.'

I'd always been a practical girl. I wore pants with pockets and cheap, comfortable tops. There's blood, vomit and bile. Even if I did own any nice clothes, I wouldn't be wearing them in the Emergency Department. But I kept my mouth shut because John was my ride back to Melbourne and I didn't intend on going back on the train with all my luggage.

11

The phone call

2011, Melbourne

Back in Melbourne, at the start of autumn I began my first
ward job as an intern on the General Medicine team. While
the other medical subspecialties look after a particular organ
system, General Medicine takes care of geriatric patients who
have co-morbidities that affect more than one system. During
this rotation, I knew the team I was on would be looking after
patients with multiple, complex conditions. A huge number
of patients was admitted under General Medicine at any one
time, so the unit was divided into three teams, each with two
interns. I was on Team B and paired with Millie from Melbourne
University, who had just finished a term as the Stroke intern.
She was already familiar with how everything worked at the
hospital, and she quickly got me up to speed. We were both
small Asian females and I wasn't convinced that people could
tell us apart, even though Millie wore contact lenses and I deliberately wore glasses to make myself look older and smarter. I'd

also started wearing a Grandpa-inspired tweed jacket now that it was getting colder in Melbourne. People often did get our names mixed up, which was annoying and a little racist, but I needed to pick my battles – it was exhausting enough doing the long ward rounds on General Medicine without getting offended or making a fuss every time someone called me 'Millie'.

We had some fantastic consultants, including the head of physician training, Professor Mary Bloom. How lucky we were to be taught and mentored by the best. The professors were all humble and insisted on being called by their first names, which felt insolent to the Japanese girl inside me, who would never call a senior colleague without their designation. It was a contrast to what I knew of the surgeons in Melbourne, who were even more formal than their Sydney counterparts: instead of 'Dr' their titles reverted to 'Mr' or 'Ms' after specialisation, like they do in England. Historically, surgeons trained under an apprenticeship model rather than through university, so in some places they're not called doctors.

Even now, I'm still unsure as to whether I completely understood everything that was going on with each patient on my General Medicine rotation. A few cases especially have stuck in my mind. We had a patient called Mrs Vasilakis, who came in with a fever of unknown origin. As part of the investigations, my registrar, Anna, asked me to refer Mrs Vasilakis to Cardiology for a transoesophageal echo – an ultrasound scan to look at her heart.

'Hello, it's Ray,' picked up the cardiology registrar.

'Oh hello, this is Yumiko, the Gen Med B intern,' I started, instantly feeling apologetic. 'I'm sorry to bother you, but may I refer a patient?'

'Sure, go ahead,' he replied, as I frantically gathered all my notes for Mrs Vasilakis, while telling Ray her full name and medical record number.

'Mrs Vasilakis is an eighty-four-year-old lady with fever of unknown origin for the past three weeks. She has been otherwise asymptomatic, but has raised inflammatory markers. She has a history of diabetes, osteoarthritis, and an artificial heart valve —'

'Stop right there,' said Ray. I stopped, a bit surprised by the interruption. 'You should have told me about her valve at the start of the referral. If you want to get the attention of a cardiology registrar, start with that information first,' he said.

It was a good piece of advice. Even though Ray came across as abrupt, I realised he was being kind by giving me feedback on my referral. I quickly learned the tips of the trade when it came to making referrals. Making consistently good referrals meant that registrars trusted you and didn't feel the need to grill you.

The number of patients on our ward increased as the weather got colder – there was always a peak in hospital admissions during winter because of respiratory illnesses. The ward rounds grew increasingly long and I felt like I was running endlessly around the hospital doing tasks for each patient, getting paged for the next task before I could finish the previous one. During one hectic ward round, my mobile phone rang in my pocket. Dad. Why was he calling me now? I got a bit frustrated. My family knew I was a doctor. Why would they interrupt me when I was working? I had seniors to impress and a ward round to follow. I was determined to get full marks for every single rotation.

When we reached the next cubicle, my phone rang once more. Dad again.

'Do you need to get that?' asked Anna.

'No, it's just my dad. Sorry,' I said in a fluster, trying to balance four folders on one arm and carrying my clipboard in the other.

Hajime was in Japan on a business trip, and had taken some time while he was there to visit his parents. Had he got the time difference wrong? Irritated, I switched my mobile to 'silent' and continued the ward round, which lasted all day. Millie and I took turns: one of us would do tasks for one set of patients while the other followed the ward round to take down the tasks needed for the second set. Our tag team was smooth and seamless, and we managed to finish the round and do all of our tasks by 6 pm. As interns we were only rostered until 4 pm and we were discouraged from claiming any overtime because we were expected to be able to finish everything we needed to do within paid hours. If you were to take two hours more than you had rostered, the thinking was that you were inefficient.

When I got home I finally looked again at my phone and found a few more missed calls from my father, and a voice message. 'Yumiko. Ji-chan's died . . .' Dad's voice trailed off.

Fuck. I called Dad back immediately but it went to his voice message. I was distraught; tears of regret were falling down my face and forming stains of shame on my blouse. *I'm so sorry, Dad. I'm sorry for being pissed off at you for calling. I'm sorry that you couldn't get through when you desperately wanted to. Most of all, I'm sorry, Grandpa.*

Ji-chan had smoked for most of his adult life. He'd had bypass surgery for a heart attack several years before but he'd bounced back and was doing fine. Hajime certainly wasn't expecting Ji-chan's rapid deterioration: Grandpa had been rushed to the Intensive Care Unit of the local hospital in Matsuyama after he began running out of air. The doctors there tried everything, but they were unable to help him. Grandpa knew he was dying, so he told my father that he was proud of all of us, and asked him to put us on the phone one by one. His lungs were so stiff that they couldn't be ventilated, but with the air he still had left he wanted to talk to us. But he didn't get to talk to me, and that's something I'll carry with me forever. I felt the most terrible daughter and an even worse granddaughter. I vowed never to ignore phone calls from family again. Sure, I'd become a doctor thinking I would put Medicine before all else: knife before life. But, really, how stupid. I'd never get that final chat with Ji-chan.

That night I opened the camera roll on my phone and looked at the last selfie I'd taken with my grandfather. We were both making silly faces. I laughed. And then I cried. Life is so fragile.

I suddenly felt really isolated, living in Melbourne with two relative strangers. I hated that I wasn't with my family, even though I knew we probably wouldn't have talked about Ji-chan's death even if I had been in Sydney. Japanese people don't do that, we move on. But being physically there would have been better. One thing I was glad about was that Ji-chan had managed to talk to my sisters. But I continued to feel dreadfully guilty that he hadn't been able to reach me, his fellow Rabbit.

Back on the wards it was becoming clear to me that the male interns were having an easier time of it than us girls, and particularly the good-looking male interns. Carlos, for example, was the centre of the nurses' gossip on the General Medicine ward. He was a handsome half-Spanish, half-Malaysian intern from Melbourne who rode a motorcycle to and from work. Every morning as he walked in wearing his leather jacket, you could see the gaze of every young female nurse following. Could the cliché of the nurse–doctor flirtation be unfolding in front of me?

'Is Carlos single?' one of the nurses asked.

'I don't know,' I replied.

'Can you find out?' she asked.

'Sure,' I replied, wondering whether this might get me into her good books.

Carlos had no trouble at all getting nurses to do exactly as he asked. In fact, they practically fought over who would help him whenever he needed a task done. It was frustrating that, even though I was polite and warm, I didn't seem to receive the same treatment. I accepted wholly that each time I started a new term as a doctor I would have to work hard to earn the respect of my nursing colleagues. Being a good doctor wasn't enough, however: you needed to be liked. God help the doctor that the nurses don't like. How your colleagues treated you meant the difference between a good day and a bad one. But it wasn't only that you needed to be liked; it turned out that if you were nice *and* attractive, you had it made! As unfair as it seemed, *c'est la vie*.

A few weeks after Ji-chan's death my team was looking after a delightful elderly gentleman, Mr Archibald. He had severe heart failure from a problem with one of his cardiac valves. That meant his feeble heart could no longer pump blood around his body, causing fluid to leak into his lungs. He was literally drowning in his own secretions. We could give him diuretics to help his body get rid of some of that fluid, but those very diuretics were killing his kidneys. It was a double-edged sword that was stabbing his heart one way and his kidneys the other, a losing battle. How would one rather die – from heart failure or kidney failure?

Each day that went by, Mr Archibald grew more and more breathless. A delicate discussion about palliation was needed. I referred Mr Archibald to Jake, the medical registrar doing the Palliative Care rotation. Jake had an excellent reputation among the doctors. He was softly spoken with a gentle way with patients. There was something attractive about a man who was both good at his job and kind. I'd always told myself that I would be professional and not develop any romantic feelings at work, but I couldn't help my emotions. I was forming a bit of a crush on Jake.

Even though Mr Archibald's condition was completely different to my grandfather's, it made me wonder about Ji-chan's final breaths. Had he felt like he was drowning in his own pool, too? Not being able to breathe – what an awful way to die. I teared up as I thought about it, and soon the tears turned into a full-blown downpour.

'I'm sorry, Mary, can I leave the ward round for a second?' I asked. The whole team looked at me, wondering what was going on. Cheerful Yumiko was suddenly unrecognisable.

'My grandfather died a few weeks ago, and Mr Archibald reminds me of him,' I explained as I wiped my face with my sleeve.

'Oh Yumiko, why didn't you tell any of us? Go and have some tea, and take your time,' a worried Mary said, in her motherly voice.

I mouthed 'Sorry' to Millie as I left the ward round and went to make a cup of tea in the ward kitchen. It did help. There's something about feeling warm liquid go down your oesophagus, warming up your chest from the inside, that's always comforting. God, why did I have to cry? I was a little horrified and embarrassed, thinking back to the other time I'd had to excuse myself from a clinical environment, when the chemotherapy ward had reminded me of Akuto-san's death.

I held the Styrofoam cup between my two hands and took deep breaths, fighting the pressure to get back to the ward round. I knew going back straightaway was unwise – I didn't want the tears to come again. So I waited until the sadness passed and I'd calmed down sufficiently.

I ran to help cope with my grief over Ji-chan's death. By now we'd done the Run for Kids, and I decided to sign up for a half-marathon to step up from that achievement. I had felt a tremendous sense of satisfaction when I finished the Run for Kids, but even by the time I'd got home the buzz was gone and I was thinking of the next race. It was as though each time I achieved something, I needed to one-up myself. I was addicted to that finish-line feeling, but it was short-lived. I did sometimes wonder if I'd ever be satisfied. When there's always more, you feel like you're never good enough. So you keep going, striving for the next finish line. That's how I felt about work, too. I was trying hard to be the best possible intern, but how would I feel next year? I'd probably dismiss everything I'd achieved in internship because, with each year of seniority, the previous year becomes diminished, just like medical school was no big deal to me now.

12

Confidence

2011, Melbourne

My third term was in the suburbs of Melbourne, so I took the train every day. The hospital was bigger than the one on my rural posting but much smaller than our hectic city base – compared to that, working in the suburbs was like being on a resort.

On my first day, we admitted a patient with an infection in her left arm from intravenous drug use. She'd normally be treated with strong antibiotics through a drip, but no one could get the drip in. The Emergency Department had an ultrasound machine to look for veins under the skin, but even that technique had failed. Eventually this woman, Lisa, was given the drugs in tablet form instead, but that was a compromise as they weren't as strong.

'Should I try to get a cannula in?' I asked my registrar.

'Um, sure, that would be ideal, but you know that ED couldn't get one in, even with ultrasound guidance?'

'Yes, but I'm going to give it a go,' I said optimistically. I knew I was good at procedural skills, and I knew that the patient would benefit from intravenous antibiotics. I wanted badly to get that drip in. For selfish reasons – for my ego – and for unselfish reasons – so that Lisa could receive the gold-standard treatment.

I introduced myself and made acquaintances as I touched Lisa's right forearm looking for veins. I closed my eyes to see if I could palpate anything under her tough, scarred skin. There were track marks everywhere, scars that told many stories. I felt the side of her wrist for the 'intern vein', which is where most of us go when we've run out of options, but there was nothing there. I couldn't put anything into the left forearm because that was the infected side. I moved on to her feet. I thought I could faintly see some blue under the skin on her right foot.

'Please, not the foot,' pleaded Lisa.

'But Lisa, there aren't any veins anywhere else, and there's this little blue one here – can you see it?' I asked.

'Yeah, but the foot ones really hurt,' she said. I found it ironic that someone who voluntarily stabbed herself with needles to shoot up drugs would complain of needle pain.

'Okay, just let me have one attempt,' I bargained with her.

'Fine – just one. I'm sick of people jabbing me today,' she said.

I pierced Lisa's foot, and she gave a little yelp and screwed her eyes shut. My eyes widened as I saw a bit of blood flash-back shoot into a cannula. This was good. I was in the vein.

'Okay, we're in,' I said, as I tried to push the plastic cannula over the needle so I could get that, too, into her vein.

Dammit, it wasn't moving. Her skin was so tough that I couldn't get it in.

'No luck?' she asked. I looked down, as though staring at the cannula might make it move.

'I'm sorry, Lisa,' I said.

'Wait,' she said. 'Give my right arm another go. I think you were on to something there.' Normally by this point I'd have given up, but here I had the benefit of time. In the city we were under so much pressure that you needed to know when to abandon something. Since I only had a few patients to look after here, and no pending tasks, I decided I would give it one more go.

I knew I couldn't mess up this time. Lisa trusted me now. Again, I closed my eyes, I gently poked every square inch of Lisa's forearm . . . and then I felt it. The bounce. I didn't say anything. I just grabbed the cannula. I don't think I was even breathing because I didn't want any extra movements. Not a tremble was allowed. I counted down for Lisa so that she knew what was coming. Three, two, one . . . and then . . . there was the reassuring flashback.

Now for the cannula. I pushed it with my forefinger. I got it in!

I don't know who was happier, me or Lisa. We sighed together and smiled.

'Nice work,' she said.

'Thanks. That wasn't easy,' I replied.

'I know, I'm running out of veins to shoot up, you know?'

I nodded. 'Well, we can start you on some stronger antibiotics through that drip now. We'll get your infection better faster this way,' I said. I realised then that as soon as Lisa got discharged she'd be using the vein I'd found; by succeeding with my cannula, I'd just shown her a new route for the drugs. That was awkward, but I was still pleased I'd been able to help her and that our persistence had paid off.

It was now July 2011, and back in Sydney my family was getting excited about the Women's World Cup in Germany. Not many Australians I knew were into women's football (or women's sport in general) back then, and even if they were, they most certainly stopped watching after the Matildas were knocked out by Sweden in the quarter-finals. But Nadeshiko Japan was still a contender. It is an unexpected name for a football team – nadeshiko is a stringy, pink flower and also describes an idealised woman in Japan – someone who is feminine and graceful. A stark contrast to the men's team, who are called the Samurai Blue.

Nadeshiko Japan was having a spectacular tournament, defying the odds and causing an upset over their German hosts to make their first ever World Cup semi-final. It was a boost for a country that had been drowned by tragedy earlier in the year. Areas affected by the Tohoku earthquake and tsunami were still rebuilding, and the *konjo* – fighting spirit – with which the players approached each game reflected the collective resilience of Japan. The head coach, Norio Sasaki, reportedly showed the team images from the natural disaster to inspire them to 'do it for Japan'.

I put my Nadeshiko Japan jersey on, acquired and worn for this month of magnificent Japanese soccer, and video-called my family so we could watch the final together, cheering at my little screen. Japan was the underdog against the almighty

United States. With three minutes left of extra time, we were losing 1–2. The world expected the US to thrash Japan, so this score was very respectable, and something to be proud of – for Japan even to make it to the final was brilliant. But I so badly wanted my team to win. *Do it for Japan.*

Then, well into extra time, the captain, Homare Sawa, a veteran playing in her fifth World Cup, scored the equaliser. I sat bolt upright, gripping my phone screen so hard that my fingers were white, as the tense penalty shoot-out was underway. Could Japan actually win this thing?

It was agonising to watch, and then ... Saki Kumagai scored the winning penalty and it was 3–2. Nadeshiko Japan was crowned the World Cup champions! I felt a huge lump in my throat as Sawa lifted the World Cup trophy under a cascade of gold confetti. Japan really needed this victory. Sporting triumphs like this lift the national mood. 'We did it for the people of Tohoku,' said Sawa in one of her media conferences.

The jubilation of Nadeshiko Japan's victory kept my spirits up for several days. It made me feel optimistic about the future; I felt empowered and I'd found a new role model in Sawa. She was awarded the Golden Ball *and* the Golden Boot – for being the most valuable player and the top scorer for the World Cup. It was a great moment for women in general, but seeing a Japanese woman with those accolades was even more impressive, knowing how hard it was for Japanese women to play football. Nadeshiko Japan was a talking point for Japanese people, and I knew it would elevate the status of professional women's football in the country; it hadn't really received a lot of recognition or support in the past. Many players still had to work part-time jobs while training. I'd grown up inspired by the marathon runner Yuko Arimori; now there was Homare Sawa. I wondered if I would ever find a female role model in surgery.

It was now time to start thinking about residency jobs for next year. That's the thing – people get this idea that being a doctor gives you job security, but there's no guarantee that your current place of employment will keep you on, so you have to apply for jobs every year. This time I knew that I needed to do an Intensive Care rotation because it's highly regarded in surgical applications. Also, I was genuinely interested in ICU, where you must become more confident and competent in looking after the sickest patients in the hospital – a valuable experience for any doctor.

So I was eyeing one of the eight sought-after Critical Care residency positions at my Melbourne hospital. Slowly, I was thinking about the future and what I had to do to maximise my chances of getting on to the Program for Plastics. Applying for – and winning – a Critical Care residency was the only guarantee of an ICU rotation and would be a significant boon for my Program application.

For my next term I returned to the mothership, where I was back in Emergency. Unlike other terms, there's a lot of autonomy working in Emergency. I got to assess patients and come up with a management plan on my own, rather than following a registrar on a ward round and doing as I was told, which happens on ward jobs such as Medicine and Surgery. Each time I ran my plan past an ED consultant, I knew it was an opportunity to demonstrate my clinical judgement. I could see early on that this term would give me every chance to shine.

My first patient had pain in his back and down one leg from a disc compressing a nerve. The neurosurgical registrar, Polly, happened to be nearby, so I walked up to her timidly – I still couldn't be sure how any of these registrars would respond to an intern asking them for stuff. Polly was from England. She was tall and had her blonde hair tied in a low bun. Not quite a chignon. I did notice, however, that she was wearing pearl earrings.

'Hi, are you the neurosurgical registrar?' I asked her.

'What do you need?' she huffed, without looking at me.

'I'd like to refer a patient to you,' I answered, a little disappointed by her curt response. 'He's got an exacerbation of pain from a known disc prolapse, and —'

'That's fine.' She cut me off brusquely. 'I'll add him to my list. Where is he?'

'Cubicle B14. Thank you,' I said, handing her the patient's sticker and scurrying away before she could tell me off for anything I had or hadn't done. I hid behind a large grey computer screen to see which patient was next in line to be assessed, and waited until Polly had left the area before going to see to the patient.

She was an elderly lady who needed a medical admission. That day Jake was the medical registrar taking referrals – the doctor who'd caught my eye when I was a general medicine intern and he was the palliative care registrar. I was glad to see that he was now working in ED, taking all the General Medicine referrals. I remembered how he was really nice and easy-going, so that took some of the pressure off making this next referral. After spending a lot of time on the medical wards in the previous two terms, I knew exactly how to present the patients. I knew the structure. I knew the buzz words. I wanted to impress him.

'You're pretty good at referrals,' he said, after I'd finished.

'Oh really? What do I get out of ten, Jake?' I asked, with a bit of cheek.

'Nine.'

'What?' I gasped with feigned dramatics. 'Why not ten?'

'Don't be too confident, you're still an intern,' he said with a smile, which really made his cheeks dimple. I smiled back, and went to find another patient to refer to him.

The interviews for the Critical Care residency positions came and went, and a few weeks later, I found out I'd been offered one of the spots. Not only that but the next time I bumped into Mary Bloom, she congratulated me and leaned in to whisper in my ear, 'You're not meant to know this, but you were ranked first of all the interns. I'm so proud of you.'

I was ecstatic. I thanked her profusely for the feedback, and did a little happy dance on the inside. Moments like this built me up. I was optimistic about the future. I felt like I was getting closer to my dream of becoming a surgeon. That afternoon I called my parents, and then my medical school mentor Dr Stein. 'That's fantastic!' his voice roared down the phone. He told me to come and see him when I came back to Sydney, and I promised I would do that.

The hospital held a lavish ball in the spring, which was exciting because I knew that Jake would be going. I invited Martha and Lily over for pre-drinks before we headed towards the city for the ball. I wore a long cream dress with a blush-coloured waist belt and some dangly earrings; Jake looked fresh in a crisp white shirt, skinny black tie and black suit, with his black glossy hair styled and waxed impeccably. By then I had made countless referrals to him so he knew who I was when I approached him on the dance floor. I'd had some bubbly, which made me even more outgoing than usual, and we struck up a conversation, laughed and joked, and then we danced.

After that night Jake and I started dating. Like all other doctors, it was impossible for us not to 'talk shop' all the time, but we did have other things in common, one being music. Jake was very talented at composition. Most days after work, we'd sit on the couch and he'd sing me some of the songs he wrote on his guitar. Having a man serenade me on the guitar was such a dream. Jake also enjoyed running. We were both training for the half-marathon so we often ran together after work. I was glad to have found someone who shared so many hobbies with me, feeling the best I had in a long time. Life was perfect: I'd got the job I wanted for next year, and I was dating a guy I fancied. The only thing that did bother me about the relationship was the fact that Jake wanted to keep it a secret. He was worried that he'd look predatory for dating an intern a few years his junior. There were plenty of medical couples at the hospital, so I didn't see it as an issue. It wasn't like I wanted him to announce it all over Facebook, but some acknowledgement of my existence would have been nice. I decided that it wasn't worth fighting over because things were otherwise going well. It did make me wonder how long he was planning on hiding me for, though . . .

13

Surgery

2011, Melbourne

Good things come to those who wait. The fifth and final term of my internship: my Surgical term at last. I was the intern for the Upper Gastrointestinal Surgery (UGIS) team, and I told myself that this was another chance to impress. I studied the conditions I would need to know about – gallstones, pancreatitis, liver disease. Mental preparation was important. The night before my first day with the team, I planned how I would get to the wards early, read all the notes of my new patients, familiarise myself with their history, see how they had progressed over the weekend, and jot down their observations from the nursing charts. I went to bed early, setting my alarm clock for 4 am. The next morning, to make sure I had sustenance for a potentially long day, I had eggs and spinach for breakfast, just like Popeye.

When I got to the surgical ward I printed the inpatient list for me and my new registrar, Rob. I'd noticed him around when he was seeing referrals in ED and he seemed to be well respected. There were twenty patients under our care, all with complicated conditions. As planned the night before, I made sure I knew everything I needed to know about each one. I started an entry in each of their notes: *Kadota (Intern) UGIS*. I wrote down their morning observations – heart rate, blood pressure, temperature – and then left a bit of space for scribing Rob's assessment and plan when we went on the ward round. With some time to spare, I made myself a cup of tea and waited in the registrars' office. Rob walked in casually. 'Oh, hey! You're here early. You're the new intern, right?'

'Yes, I'm Yumiko,' I said, passing him his copy of the patient list.

He looked at it. 'Promise me you won't do that again,' he said.

'Oh?' I was a little confused.

'Buddy, we're a team. We can start at the same time, no need to get here before me,' he laughed. 'Chill.'

'Okay,' I replied, knowing I would still come in early tomorrow, because that's what a good intern does.

After the ward round, there were no urgent tasks so Rob took me to a café down the road from the hospital. He bought coffees and chocolate croissants, and did the usual start-of-term chat, asking things like what terms I'd done this year, how internship was going, and what I wanted to be when I grew up.

'I want to do Surgery,' I said, confidently. *Don't be a wall-flower, Yumiko.*

'That's great!' he said. 'Do you know what kind of surgery?'

'Yes, I'm interested in Plastics, although I haven't done a term in it yet.'

'You want to come to theatre later?'

'Yes, please!' My eyes lit up.

'Awesome,' he replied. 'I could use a hand.'

'I'll get all my jobs done before then,' I said, and headed for the ward, motivated to get everything completed as soon as possible so that I could go to the operating theatre to assist Rob. I hadn't had an opportunity like this all year, so I was determined to see this one through.

Surgical registrars had a reputation for being unceremonious. They were much harder to call up than other doctors because Surgery seemed to attract people who were blunt and straight to the point. I thought of Dr Stein's registrar Ingrid and all her F-words. I guessed you had to be tough, working such long hours, and under constant time pressure. Rob wasn't like that, though. He was so cool and laidback. He must have been a mature-age student at university because he was older than the other registrars, with a wife and two young kids. How lovely to already have a family. I wouldn't have said they had it easy, though. Rob's wife was a final-year medical student so it was stressful at home with her needing to study for her exams, as well as Rob's demanding schedule. In my mind I still romanticised the idea of being a mum, but I couldn't square it with a career as a surgeon. There weren't many examples around me of female surgeons who were both at the top of their careers while successfully balancing family life. There was only one general surgeon who had a family. I'd seen her bringing her children into work when she had to do a ward round one weekend. It did make me wonder whether she had a partner, and whether they were also at work. And if so, why did this surgeon have to be the one looking after the children? All the other female consultants were single, so things didn't look too promising for my romantic future. It did play on my mind sometimes; I was well aware of the sacrifices I'd have to make in order to succeed in Surgery.

Rob was still his chirpy self as we approached 7 pm. Nothing seemed to faze him. I hoped I could be like that, too. We'd been at hospital for over twelve hours, waiting for one last emergency operation. I was meant to be having dinner with Jake, but I cancelled. I didn't even think twice about it. I promised him I'd make up for it by cooking dinner on the weekend. Was I already behaving in a way that'd put off Jake and future partners? Was this the sort of thing that eventually gnawed away at relationships? I wondered whether life as a surgical registrar would be like this – bargaining with friends and loved ones all the time – a continuous cycle of cancelling and making up for cancelling.

The patient Rob was operating on that evening had perforated his bowel and needed an urgent surgery called a Hartmann's procedure. Rob talked me through what he was doing, and I absorbed every moment, every cut and stitch. I wasn't even tired by the end of the operation, I had so much adrenaline running through me. It was worth staying back for that feeling. Besides, as an intern with future surgical aspirations, I'd have looked uninterested if I hadn't stayed.

When I got home I took a shower and lay in bed staring at the ceiling, smiling and looking forward to assisting more surgeries.

The next morning, I met a new patient, George, and his wife, Wendy. George was in his early forties and had had surgery just six weeks before for an aggressive cancer called a cholangiocarcinoma. Luckily, it had been caught early and the post-operative scan showed no sign of residual disease.

But George had started having pain again the week before, and was looking a little yellow.

'Order a scan,' instructed Rob.

I wrote it down on my to-do list.

'Make sure it happens today,' said Rob.

Our next patient on the ward round was a man with a rare condition called SMA syndrome, where the duodenum gets crushed between two arteries. He needed to go to the operating theatre to bypass this compression – a surgery I'd never seen before and was keen to experience. Jake was leaving on a flight that afternoon for a medical conference in Brisbane. After completing the morning's tasks, including ordering George's scan, I decided I'd have a coffee with Jake and walk him to the tram stop outside the hospital. It felt good to catch him before he had to leave, even though he was only going away for a few days.

He didn't want to hold hands to the tram stop because he didn't want anyone to see us, but he did allow me to give him a hug at the stop. My gut instinct was telling me that there was something wrong with all this, but I ignored it because I was smitten. I hadn't had a boyfriend in so long and I enjoyed the companionship. Having no family in Melbourne, Jake had sort of become my family. We spent as much of the week together as we could and I wanted desperately for us to work out.

When I walked back into the hospital I found out that I'd missed the surgery. I was angry with myself. Did I really need to walk Jake to the tram? He was a grown man – he could have walked himself. I'd just denied myself an opportunity to learn, an opportunity to observe how the surgeons would operate on this rare case, and for me to watch a new procedure. I was kicking myself and knew I'd regret this for weeks. I decided that I needed to keep a closer eye on what was happening in the operating theatres so that I didn't miss any more surgeries, and I began to watch the theatre list obsessively, walking past the reception every hour.

George returned to the ward from his scan. I found Rob and we looked at the images together. George's cancer was back, and so aggressively that the little seed that must have been left behind at the time of his operation had spread wildly in the few weeks that he'd been back at home. 'Shit,' muttered Rob. The cancer did not look operable. He rang the consultant straightaway, who confirmed that there was nothing more we could do for George.

Rob went to deliver the bad news, and asked that I get George's discharge papers ready and make a referral to Oncology and Palliative Care. I nodded. Words couldn't come out of my mouth, I was so devastated. I made some phone calls and wrote letters for George to bring to his appointments, and went to give them to him. He was sitting up in bed, with Wendy perched on the end.

'Hi, Yumiko,' they said in unison, as I approached the bed-side. I drew the curtains around his cubicle for some privacy.

'As Rob would have explained, I've made some referrals.' I handed over the letters.

'Thank you,' he said. This man had inoperable cancer and he was thanking me? I couldn't bear it. I felt that ominous lump in my throat. I looked up at the ceiling to try to stop the tears that were starting to form.

'I'm so sorry that the cancer's returned,' I said in a husky voice, feeling my throat constricting and a hot swelling build inside my nose. Before I knew it, I was crying. *Oh no.* I looked at George, and then at Wendy.

'I'm so sorry. This is so unprofessional, I'm sorry. You can report me to the Medical Board,' I said, choking on my tears.

'Don't be silly,' Wendy reassured me. 'Thank you for caring.'

George was the one with the cancer invading his body, yet it was his wife who was comforting me. This wasn't how it was meant to go. I excused myself to blow my nose, wash my face and calm myself down. In the ward kitchen I made two cups of tea and brought them to George and Wendy. It felt such a helpless situation, and if I couldn't do anything medically, at least tea was comfort in a mug, and it was something small I could offer.

'Would you like milk or sugar with your tea?' I asked George.

'Fuck it, I'm dying. Load it up with sugar!' he said. We all laughed. Even after being delivered the worst possible news, George could still crack a joke. That made me cry even more.

'I'm not dying, but fuck it, I'll have sugar too,' said Wendy.

'Done. Here you go,' I said, passing their cups over. 'Dilmah tea. The hospital's finest.'

'Thanks, champ,' he said. The lovely couple smiled at me sympathetically. In that moment, the barriers blurred: I was not their doctor but simply a fellow human.

'I'll give you some privacy,' I said, stepping back. 'I'm sorry again for the bad news, and I'm sorry for getting emotional.'

14

Canary in a coalmine

2012, Melbourne

My left hand was cramping from writing in my diary. It was the last day of internship and there was so much to reflect on. What a massive year. On my rural placement I'd faced the thing I feared the most – death. And I lost Ji-chan not long after that. George was still on my mind, too – I wondered how he was doing. As doctors we spend our years studying diseases and how to manage them, but there's still so much we can't do. We don't have a cure for cancer. Sometimes, I realised, the most important thing I could do as a doctor was to be kind.

Just before Christmas, Jake's parents visited him and we met at a restaurant. I was keen to make a good impression. I wore my best version of a 'meet the parents' outfit – a simple black jacquard dress to the knee and some sensible black kitten heels – straightened my hair and wore some pearl earrings. Jake's parents were delightful. As soon as they saw me, they gave me a warm hug. The conversation flowed seamlessly over dinner and they commented on how great the chemistry was between me and Jake. At the end of the night they asked if I'd like to join them the next morning for breakfast; I took that to mean that the first impression was good. Maybe it was the pearl earrings.

I flew back to Sydney for Christmas, and Jake joined me a week later for New Year's. After the success of meeting his parents, I was excited for him to meet mine and hoped they would love him as much as I did. We decided to meet over yum cha at a local Chinese restaurant. Jake was running late and waiting for him I was jittery, nervously spinning the lazy Susan around. He eventually arrived and sat down next to me. I could tell that he was trying earnestly to build rapport with my parents, but the conversation kept stalling. It was worse than the time he'd tried to teach me how to drive a manual. I looked over at my sisters, who looked disengaged. After lunch, when we'd got home, I asked Yoshiko what she thought of Jake. She said, 'He seems selfish.'

In January 2012 I started my year as a Critical Care resident, which was more formally known as a 'house medical officer 2'. 'Kadota – HMO2'. It felt good writing that on the medical charts. I was so ready to be a resident; I was sick of writing 'Intern' – it made me feel like a trainee at McDonald's.

My first term of the year was in Neurosurgery. Some of us were rotating through Cardiothoracic Surgery, while others of us were assigned to Neurosurgery – these were the two surgical specialties at the hospital that looked after critically unwell patients. I was a bit nervous because one of my seniors would be neurosurgical registrar Polly, with whom I'd had that encounter in the Emergency Department. As it turned out, when we came across one another she was friendly and didn't seem to clock that she'd ever laid eyes on me before, let alone snapped at me.

Polly had moved to Australia from Norfolk in England, where she'd worked in the National Health Service. The NHS simply couldn't offer enough job security, and many of its doctors felt they weren't being looked after by the system, they weren't valued or respected, and the teams within which they worked were deeply demoralised. Years later, the exodus from the NHS and British medicine came to be known as the Drexit. Those who left tended to either retrain in new professions, or head to Australia, New Zealand or Canada, which had reputations for being better-run systems and offering more stability for doctors. Better how, I didn't know – I hadn't worked anywhere else for comparison. Besides, I'd only worked for a year as an intern. So far, I'd enjoyed my time as a doctor in Melbourne and hoped that it would continue to be this way. I mean, if these doctors were moving all the way to Australia, we must really have it good here.

On my first day I met Charlie, another resident. Charlie was new to the hospital. She was born and raised in Australia, but her background was Laotian. She had completed medical school, internship and residency in Tasmania, but wanted the experience of working in a major trauma centre. She walked over to join the rest of us for the ward round. Charlie was also interested in Plastic Surgery, and we immediately bonded over that. I got a warm vibe from her and I was sure we were going to have a good term working together.

By lunchtime we had finished our tasks, so I suggested to Charlie that we grab some food and eat in the common room – the residents' quarters, or 'ressies', as they were more affectionately known. But Charlie thought we should stay close to the ward just in case the registrars needed us.

'Charlie, that's what pagers are for,' I said. 'If they need us, they'll page.'

'Nah, it's cool. Maybe we can eat at the café today.'

'Ressies is more comfortable,' I suggested. 'Come on, let's go.'

'I can't.'

'What do you mean?'

'I don't want to go to the ressies. My cousin committed suicide there.'

Oh god, I felt terrible and immediately wished I'd kept quiet.

'It was a while ago, when I was a second-year med student,' Charlie said. 'I went to his funeral, but no one spoke about it. You know what Asian families are like.'

Charlie told me her cousin's story. Loy was a surgical registrar who was very close to finishing his specialist training. But his on-call roster was brutal and he had been working excessive hours – his shifts were reportedly twenty-four to thirty-six hours long. On top of the heavy workload he had the pressure of exams, which he needed to pass to progress to the next stage, the summit: consultant. He was sleep deprived and overworked. Eventually, he couldn't take it anymore. Loy took a lethal dose of medications in ressies and was unable to be revived.

The story was devastating. I knew about suicides in the medical profession, but this was the first time I'd ever spoken to someone who'd been directly affected. It shook me to the core.

Doctors not only have the knowledge about which drugs can kill you, and how many to take, but they have access to the drugs, too. I wondered whether the hospital had altered the registrar rostering after Loy's death, or whether – like all other doctor suicides, it seemed – they chose to see it as an isolated, tragic case.

Suicide was something I had heard about at medical school but never discussed with any of my fellow students. We just didn't talk about mental health. A couple of my friends had shared with me that they were taking antidepressants, but that was the extent to which I'd engaged on this topic. To be honest, I'd always had the 'it won't happen to me' mentality, so perhaps it was due to my own ignorance that I knew nothing more about the insidiousness of mental illness plaguing the medical community. I knew that mental illness could affect anyone, but I felt secure in that I had a lot of protective factors. There was no history of mental illness in my family, I was physically healthy, I exercised a lot, and I was privileged to have received a good education and to have a great job. I knew that these factors made me less vulnerable to mental illness.

Charlie was newly single after breaking up with her girlfriend recently. I spoke to her about Jake, who was taking 2012 off to travel. I loved the idea of travelling the world with him, but the timing wasn't right. After only a year of internship and having succeeded in achieving my hard-fought Critical Care placement, leaving the workforce now would be a poor decision. Initially, Jake wanted me to remain his girlfriend, but after a while we realised that long distance wasn't going to work for us. Actually, if I was being brutally honest with myself, 'us' meant 'him'. Jake wanted to be single while he was travelling, so he broke up with me – via email. Perhaps Yoshiko was right – mums do have an instinct about these things – maybe he was selfish. Still, even though I was heartachingly disappointed, I needed to refocus. I'd hoped very much that Jake loved me enough to continue the relationship, but I knew I needed to move on. Dabbing away the tears that dripped off my chin, I walked around my room pulling out the weeds of our relationship – cards, presents, some socks he'd left behind. I wasn't quite ready to let them go, but I didn't want any reminders of Jake, so I put the relics in an old shoebox to give to Martha for safekeeping. Out of sight, out of mind.

Now was the time to start work in earnest on my application for the Program. It would still be a few years before I would officially apply, but it was never too early to begin preparing and laying the groundwork. After internship and residency, the ideal path for a doctor is to spend a limited time as an unaccredited registrar before winning a spot on a training program to gain experience in a chosen specialty. But there are only a limited number of spots on the Program each year, so some doctors spend years and years as an 'unaccredited' registrar before they're able to become 'accredited' by getting on to the Program. There's a risk that you'll never make it on there, of course, so you could potentially spend an endless number of precious years in the position of being unaccredited. In that case, there are only two options: you give up, or you keep going until you do get on.

Candidates were short-listed for interview based on their CV and referees. I still hadn't done a Plastic Surgery term as a resident so I didn't have any references yet – they would come next year. However, I was working hard on scoring as many points as possible for my CV. I had already completed a surgical literature course, which counted for a few points, and that weekend I was doing a surgical skills course at the College of Surgeons.

Anushka, a senior registrar in Neurosurgery, had been accepted on to the training program as a young resident, and was already in her third year of training. She was a superstar at the hospital. Most doctors take a few attempts to get on to the Program, but she'd been accepted on her first try, which made her stand out. I hoped I could be like her.

As Charlie and I were talking about our love lives, she came to join us for lunch.

'How are you finding the hospital?' she asked me.

'I love it!' I exclaimed. 'I had such a great internship.'

'It's a lot better than where I last worked,' she said.

'Why's that?' asked Charlie.

'The consultants were savage,' Anushka said. 'I once got told off in theatre and the boss stomped on my foot . . . and it broke!'

'What? Are you serious?' I was in disbelief.

'Yeah. That sort of thing happens all the time in surgery.'

'I can't believe he broke your foot!' I said. 'Did you report him?'

'I couldn't. You can't. You'll get kicked off the Program.'

'That's crap,' Charlie chimed in. 'Surgeons get away with so much.'

'I'm shocked,' I said. 'I mean, I've heard of surgeons throwing scalpels and instruments on the floor, but breaking your foot?'

'That's assault,' Charlie said.

Our conversation abruptly halted with the sound of the pager. MET call. Medical emergency team. The three of us rushed back to the ward. One of our patients was losing consciousness. He'd had surgery the day before to insert a drain called an EVD that was draining fluid from the ventricles inside his brain. Anushka took charge of the situation. She was calm and clear in her instructions. She adjusted the height of the EVD to change its drainage as I stood back and observed the situation, documenting everything in the notes. The patient started to pick up.

Anushka left the ward to inform the consultant, Professor Kaufmann, of what had happened. I finished writing in the patient's notes and sat at the computer station on the ward for a while longer. My heart was beating fast. Neurosurgery was scary. The patients can deteriorate quickly, and the brain is so complex. It was intimidating. And what was with that foot stomping? I was starting to see how sinister surgery could be. I wondered how I would react if someone injured my foot on purpose. I just hoped I would never find myself in that sort of situation. It seemed such an extreme incident that I reassured myself it was unlikely anything like that would happen to me.

'Oh look, it's the Powerpuff Girls,' said a tall man who'd just walked on to the ward.

'This is Prof Kaufmann,' said Anushka, who was with him.

'Who is this?' he asked, pointing at me.

'That's Yumiko, one of our new residents.'

'Ah, Cherry Blossom,' he said, and offered his hand. 'Welcome to Neurosurgery. The best of all the surgical specialties!'

I smiled awkwardly and shook his hand.

'*Nuide kudasai*,' he said. 'Take off your clothes' in Japanese. He gave a loud belly laugh. I quietly laughed along with him to be polite. I thought to myself, *what a creep*, but I wasn't going to say that out loud – he was the clinical director of Neurosurgery, after all. He took me, Charlie and Anushka into a cubicle to talk to a thirty-five-year-old woman who had an aneurysm in her brain.

'Hello. I am Professor Kaufmann,' he said in a booming, deep voice. 'You have an aneurysm, which I would recommend surgery for. You know what an aneurysm is?'

'Yes, your registrars —'

'An aneurysm is like a nipple. You know, tits are great, but not this kind of tit,' explained Prof Kaufmann. I looked over at Anushka, my mouth gaping, eyes wide. Did he really just say that? Anushka stood there, expressionless, like she had heard it all before.

As he left the ward, Prof Kaufmann looked at me and Charlie. 'You only have to remember one thing this term,' he said, raising his pointer finger to the roof. 'I am God on this ward.'

Despite Kaufmann's bedside manner, the patient agreed to have an elective clipping of her aneurysm. Unfortunately she developed a complication after surgery – a stroke. There was this young, beautiful lady limping around the ward with a walking stick, completely aphasic – she could not speak at all. She worked really hard with the speech pathologist but she barely regained her speech. I referred her to rehab, knowing that she would be there for a long time before she could walk or talk properly. I was gutted. I was gutted for her and the result she got, and I was gutted about how she had been spoken to at that first consultation. I asked Anushka about it. She said that she was used to it; her attitude to it was a 'boys will be boys' kind of thing. As we spoke, she took off her thick-rimmed glasses and rubbed her eyes. She looked weary and said she hadn't washed her hair in a week. Perhaps she was too tired from her registrar responsibilities to get outraged about anything.

Towards the end of the Neurosurgery term, the Summer Olympics kicked off in London and the Japanese Football Association (JFA) made the news. The World Cup–winning women's team, Nadeshiko Japan, was flown in cattle class while the less successful men's team was flown business. The JFA was criticised heavily for sexism: their reasoning was that the men were professional and the women were amateur players, but this only highlighted why women weren't able to play professionally in the first place. It was hard to believe, but even after their World Cup success the women's game still didn't have the appropriate levels of support or sponsorship.

At the Games both teams did well. The men placed fourth and the women brought home the silver medal. After this result, the JFA decided to upgrade Nadeshiko Japan to business.

I talked about it with Charlie at work the next day – why Asian countries were so patriarchal. There were a few things about Japan that bothered me. One was gender inequity and the other was the lack of conversation around mental health. Charlie was a part of the Hmong community, which I didn't know much about, so I was intrigued to hear how they dealt with mental health issues.

'No one talks about mental health,' she said. I nodded in recognition. 'We have a shaman do these soul-calling ceremonies, though.'

'Soul calling?' I asked.

'Yes. When people are sick, it's thought to be because the soul has wandered,' explained Charlie. 'The shaman performs a spiritual ceremony to get the soul back, and to get rid of bad spirits. It's attended by friends and family to try to cheer up the person who's having a bit of a hard time.'

'Oh, that sounds really nice,' I said. 'It's great when the community comes together like that.'

'Do you have anything like that in Japan?' Charlie asked.

'Not that I'm aware of,' I replied.

'So anyway, we never know what exactly the problem is, but whenever someone has lots of visits from the shaman, we know something must be up.'

'So, even though no one says anything explicitly, you kind of know that there could be some mental health issues?'

'Yes, exactly.'

I went up to ressies to eat my lunch. I thought about Charlie's cousin and wondered whether there had been any warning signs that Loy was distressed. Had the shaman been called to see him before he died? The canary in the coalmine. Surgical registrars are known to be tough – the workload really must have been excessive for him to have gone to that very dark place. Poor Loy. I thought about what had changed since then. At least they locked up anaesthetic drugs to make it harder for people to access them. But did that address the underlying issue? The fact that surgical registrars had these gruelling on-call rosters made me a little nervous. I knew I had to brace myself for this precarious coalmine. As I worked on my Program application, I hoped that I would never be pushed to that extreme.

15

Nights

2012, Melbourne

After my Neurosurgery term, I did a term in Intensive Care. The arrangement of staff in the ICU was completely different. Firstly, the registrars and consultants rotated every week, so I was working with a different team each time. I really missed being a part of the same team every day. I missed Charlie, Polly and Anushka – I had enjoyed having female colleagues who were also surgically minded because there weren't that many of us. Over the previous term Anushka and Polly had become my friends, as well as colleagues I respected and admired. I continued to want to emulate Anushka, and I began to understand Polly better. She was passionate and that sometimes made her impatient and hot-headed. She was the oldest of three girls, like me, and when she was just six years old one of her sisters, Harriet, had suffered a terrible accident falling off a horse. She presented to a small rural hospital in Norfolk and was found to have an extradural haemorrhage – catastrophic bleeding

140

around her brain. A general surgeon in the hospital drilled an emergency burr hole into her skull to let out the blood, but didn't consult with a neurosurgeon. Unfortunately, the procedure was inadequate and Harriet started having seizures. By the time she was transferred to a neurosurgical unit in London, she had suffered a massive stroke, which caused permanent damage.

The grief of their young daughter developing a severe brain injury and the stress of looking after a child with a disability put a lot of strain on Polly's parents, who separated just a few years later. Having experienced this family tragedy at such a young age, Polly always fought hard for her neurosurgical patients. She was one of the few doctors I knew who had a personal story that had profoundly influenced her choices and dedication to her specialty.

In contrast, I barely got to know any of the doctors in the ICU. Usually I'd be able to work out how a consultant liked things done, but in this rotation it was much harder to do that, and therefore to be able to impress the senior staff, because each of their expectations was different. What one consultant liked, another would not. I realised quickly I'd have to become super-flexible in ICU because every week I'd be working with new registrars and consultants who had their own unique way of doing things.

The second thing I came to realise about ICU was that these doctors thought that anyone doing or interested in surgery wasn't worth bothering with. There can be so much ego in a hospital – some specialties thinking they are better than the others, and in this ICU the disdain towards us surgical types was palpable. To these intensive care doctors, surgeons were just glorified carpenters. No brains, just dexterity. There's no question that Intensive Care doctors are very knowledgeable. They have the sickest patients in the hospital, who often have multiple, complex and very serious problems. Unfortunately, the knowledge of the consultants and registrars didn't necessarily make them good teachers and supervisors, or very pleasant to work with.

One week, I was under the supervision of consultant Bridget and senior registrar Donal. Bridget was always complaining. She'd bitch about the registrar who had worked the night before, unfairly criticising the choices that had been made. How about feeding this back directly to the registrar concerned rather than complaining about it to us? I had been a multitasker since my first internship rotation, completing tasks on the go to make sure I was being efficient. Bridget did not like this at all. Instead of her telling me, though, she got Donal to do so.

Donal was a big bloke with the waist circumference of an SUV tyre, and sometimes I did think about rolling him down a dirt hill. He towered over me and pointed his fat forefinger in my face one morning. 'You need to stop running off! Where do you keep going? You need to follow the ward round!' he bellowed. This large man was standing uncomfortably close to me.

'Sorry, I was just making a referral for the last patient so that it doesn't get delayed,' I tried to explain.

'No. You need to pay attention.' He was pointing his finger at my face one more time as he said 'You.' I drew back because his finger was so close to my nose. My skin started to feel a bit clammy, like a rash might be developing on my neck.

I was trying so hard to be a good resident yet I was getting reprimanded in a humiliating way. I felt like I couldn't do anything to please Bridget and Donal, even when I tried to explain why I was doing things the way I was. It was the first time I'd experienced such scrutiny about my ward work, which had been very autonomous in previous terms. I would complete tasks during the ward round because I didn't want to delay treatment for the patients. As long as the work was done, my former registrars and consultants were happy. Bridget and Donal preferred that I didn't work in this way, micro-managing everything I did. Really, I felt, I'd need to be a puppet to survive the week with them. And finding myself without a sense of ownership over my role, I felt my interest dwindling – even on that first day I began to feel disconnected from my work.

For the remainder of the week I stuck carefully to the ward round, even if it meant I couldn't get the tasks for each patient done until much later in the morning. My heart rate seemed perpetually elevated and my body felt like it was always on stand-by, ready for Donal's next attack. It was stressful not being able to predict how he and Bridget would like things done and I kept second-guessing myself, which was unlike me – until this term I had been confident in how I approached my daily tasks. It was all a bit deflating.

After the week with Bridget and Donal, I attended a two-day surgical course, a welcome relief. It was on the emergency management of severe trauma. One of the activities was learning to put a chest drain in and it felt good to learn some new practical skills and use my hands again. More importantly, it was another surgical course that would count towards the Program.

Back at work I had a new team, so I immediately abandoned Bridget's and Donal's methods and decided to be a blank canvas, awaiting instruction from my new seniors. In this second week I was working with a senior registrar, Borsi, and a junior registrar called Liam. They both knew I was interested in surgery so they didn't expect much of me. Borsi loved to ask the most esoteric of questions that no one could answer so he could sound smart, and he loved asking about the 'zebras', the rare conditions.

'So, Liam,' gleamed Borsi, turning to the junior registrar. 'This patient here has an adrenal haemorrhage. Do you know the syndrome where you have bilateral adrenal haemorrhages associated with meningococcal infection?'

'Umm, no idea,' replied Liam.

'I don't suppose you know,' Borsi said to me condescendingly.

'Waterhouse-Friderichsen syndrome,' I shot back, with a straight face.

Borsi was dumbfounded that the surgical wannabe had managed to spoil his game. He feigned a smile and we moved on. He didn't ask any more questions for the rest of the ward round and I went home on time that day.

After my twelve-week rotation in Intensive Care, I moved on to night shifts in Emergency. I had learned a lot of valuable skills, but some of the doctors in the ICU were so obnoxious that I couldn't have been happier leaving, even if my new term was made up of nights. I'd got what I needed out of the ICU term, and that's all that mattered. Box ticked. Thank you, next.

Night shifts were hard on the brain because it's unnatural for humans to be nocturnal, but there were some perks. I liked the smaller team at night. There were fewer staff members rostered on, which meant that you got to know everyone well. There was a camaraderie that didn't exist on day shifts. I noticed that the nurses brought in food to share and I liked that community feeling. The pervasive thought I had every term was that I needed the nurses on side. By this stage, I was becoming more confident as a doctor. I was hard-working and competent. But I felt like this wasn't enough. I thought that maybe bringing food to my shift would help, especially if it was something I'd made myself, so that's when I started baking before work. I never noticed male doctors bringing anything in to share. They didn't have to. For me? Cupcakes were my currency. I wasn't intentionally trying to food-bribe anyone, but I did notice that bonding over baking recipes helped me to fit in with the nurses.

What I didn't like about night shifts was having to wake up on-call registrars. Some specialties had a registrar rostered on for the night shift, but others had registrars who were on-call for twenty-four hours. That meant they worked a full day, and even after they got home they were still on stand-by for the rest of the full twenty-four-hour period. For years it was an unwritten rule that you shouldn't ring on-call doctors unless it was really urgent – no one wants to be woken up in the middle of the night unless it's an emergency. Yet this professional courtesy seemed to have become diluted with the advent of the '4-hour rule', which had just been set for Australian Emergency Departments in response to concerns that long stays in the ED meant higher death rates. The intention was to roll out the rule through each state and territory in the next few years. It stipu-lated that a patient had to be assessed and managed within four hours of arriving in ED – either they must be fully treated and discharged home or admitted to the hospital with an ongoing management plan. In theory it sounded great because patients would be seen in a timely manner. The reality was that some Emergency doctors were too keen to get patients out of the ED at the expense of thoroughly assessing them. The result was specialty registrars getting called about patients who had not been properly diagnosed.

One night I saw a patient with dizziness. He had a problem with his inner ear and would need follow up at the Vestibular Clinic, run by the ear, nose and throat surgeons. It was 1 am. This was hardly an emergency so I planned on calling the ENT registrar in the morning to make the referral. I reported back to the senior Emergency registrar Elijah to tell him my plan for the patient.

'No,' said Elijah. 'Call ENT now.'

'It's one a.m.,' I said. 'Maybe I should call him in the morning?'

'Just call – it's only one.'

Reluctantly, I walked back to my work station and picked up the phone. I really did not want to wake up the ENT registrar. I looked at the on-call roster. ENT: Lachlan. Surgical registrars start work early and regularly finish late. I didn't want to be the one who ruined Lachlan's sleep and caused him to be tired the next day. I had this awful, sinking feeling in my stomach as I waited for the hospital switchboard to pick up. The operator put me through to Lachlan's phone. He picked up in a croaky, sleepy voice. I'd woken him up. I felt guilty as I made the referral, even though Lachlan was nice about it.

Not all registrars were as tolerant. Later that year, I was covering the surgical wards at night. I attended a MET call on the ward for a patient, Mr Withey, admitted under the Vascular Surgery team. A familiar face turned up – Borsi, who was covering MET calls. Mr Withey had had surgery in the previous week and developed a droop to his face. He was having a stroke. Borsi instructed me to call the vascular registrar. It was midnight, but this time I didn't feel guilty about calling because it was a true emergency. I needed to know whether we could give Mr Withey anticoagulants for the stroke. It was a tricky conundrum that no junior doctor would decide without consulting the surgical team. Anticoagulation is needed to treat a stroke, but it increases the risk of bleeding in someone who has recently had surgery. Confident that I had a reasonable, valid question to ask, I waited on the line.

'Hello? It's Bob,' said a gruff voice.

'Hi Bob, sorry to call you so late, this is Yumiko, the night resident,' I said. 'I'd like to talk to you about Mr Withey. He's had a stroke.'

'Why are you calling me at midnight?' screamed Bob.

'I need to ask you about anticoagulation,' I replied, spooked by how irate he was.

'He had bleeding issues immediately post-op – of course he can't!' he yelled.

'Okay,' I said calmly. 'That's all I needed to know.'

The ward was silent except for the occasional bleep of monitors. I could feel the pounding of my heart in my ears. I didn't deserve to be spoken to like that. If a patient of mine had a stroke, I would want to know. Wouldn't he? Or did Bob not care? I tried not to get wound up about it. I opened Mr Withey's file on the computer and documented the event, and the instruction Bob had given before he hung up. The pager beeped as I stood up from the desk – another MET call on the other side of the ward.

Borsi was already there. This time, an elderly woman was having breathing difficulties and deteriorating quite rapidly. I took some blood from her and ordered an urgent X-ray. Then I saw the label above her bed: Vascular Surgery. I wanted to whimper. *Please, don't make me call Bob again.* Borsi and I looked through the patient's chart and found that a consultant surgeon called Mr Chandra had operated on this lady.

'Can you call Mr Chandra?' Borsi asked me.

'What do you want me to say?' I asked.

'Tell him that she is unlikely to make it to the morning,' he said.

'Okay,' I agreed reluctantly. Borsi was making me do his dirty work. No one wants to bother a consultant in the middle of the night, so with something as serious as this it was usually the most senior person in the medical emergency team who should be picking up the phone. It's a lot easier for a senior clinician to ring another senior clinician, because they have more authority. To make the junior resident, and one who barely knew the patient, call the consultant seemed unprofessional and cruel.

I rang the switchboard and asked to be put through to Mr Chandra. It was now nearly one in the morning and Mr Chandra was not impressed.

'Who are you?' he demanded.

'I'm Yumiko, the night resident.'

'The night resident!' he repeated in exasperation. 'Why is the *night resident* calling me in the middle of the night?'

I paused. This was a rhetorical question, right?

'Why are you calling me?' he pressed.

'I'm sorry. This is a courtesy call to inform you that your patient has had a MET call and is extremely unwell. She is unlikely to survive the night,' I said, trying to be brave.

'It's one o'clock in the morning! I'm not even the on-call consultant. You need to call the on-call registrar, who will then inform the on-call consultant if necessary,' he yelled and hung up the phone.

My hand felt heavy as I dropped the phone on the receiver. Two angry phone calls, one after the other. From my limited experience, it seemed as though surgeons were an apoplectic mob. I was shaken. Was it always going to be like this?

16

Human stories

2012, Melbourne

In October 2012, I was back on the Neurosurgical ward again. I was glad that I had another rotation on Neurosurgery because I liked Polly and Anushka, and they gave me hope that women could succeed in surgery. On my second day back with the Neurosurgery girls, Julia Gillard, our first female prime minister – a fact that swathes of Australia seemed not to be dealing with – made her now famous speech chastising opposition leader Tony Abbott for his misogynistic and sexist behaviours. It was such a girl-power moment to see a female politician stand up for herself in that impassioned and articulate way. I don't know how she kept herself together. Imagine facing a man who'd rallied against you in front of a 'Ditch the Witch' sign. I wanted to cry and clap at the same time. Polly spoke about it for days. 'Julia Gillard is such a badass!' she said.

One of my most memorable patients on this rotation was a man in his seventies called Oliver, who had presented with a paralysed left arm. He underwent various investigations, which showed that there was cancer growing in the brachial plexus – the nerves supplying his upper limb. A biopsy showed it was melanoma but the original melanoma was never found. After examining further scans of his body we could see that the melanoma had gone to his brain, which is when our team got involved. Oliver lived alone at home, but he had a son who sometimes came to visit. One afternoon, when I stepped outside the hospital to get some takeaway Nando's for my team, I saw him sitting on a bench outside. He looked miserable.

'Are you all right, Oliver?' I asked.

'Yeah,' he replied, and took a protracted drag from his cigarette.

We both knew he was dying. In that moment, I decided that the only thing I could really do was give him my time. I sat next to him on the bench and he talked to me about his son. He was worried about him because he'd lost his job and was struggling to pay child support. I sat there listening. We often got so caught up in the chaos on the wards that we didn't have chats with our patients. Every human has a story, and Oliver taught me that I could be a better doctor by simply listening, and caring.

As I said goodbye to Oliver and left him on the bench outside, Polly rang and asked me to join her in the ED for a new admission. When I got there, she was having a conniption at the nurse in charge. The nurse had tears in her eyes as Polly berated her in the middle of the work station for all to see. Polly was so incensed that the veins in her neck and temples were bulging, and her skin was hot-pink with rage.

'Are you an idiot? How can you transfer the patient to Short Stay? He has a large subdural haemorrhage! How can you call yourself a nurse? He needs to be monitored. Transfer him back to a main cubicle,' her voice accelerating and amplifying.

I walked up to Polly, hoping she'd see me and use that as a cue to quieten down.

'Oh, hi Miko,' she said, and walked away from the nurse, to my relief.

'Are you okay?' I asked Polly. 'Should we talk outside?'

'Yes, I'll fill you in,' she said as we walked out of the Emergency Department.

Polly's passion was what I admired most about her, but it was also the characteristic that made me nervous for her. This wasn't the first time she'd lost her temper with another staff member. I knew the pattern by now. The incident would likely be reported to the department of Neurosurgery, Polly would get called to a disciplinary meeting with Professor Kaufmann and she would have to apologise to the nurse.

Polly let off steam. Yes, I was her junior, but because we had become friends I felt comfortable telling her to rein it in.

'I can't believe that nurse is so stupid!' she carried on. 'They don't have enough staff in Short Stay to observe the patients!'

'I know,' I said. 'Moving that patient was the wrong decision . . . but you can't scream at people at work.'

'That patient could've died!'

'I know, Polly, but did you see the nurse? She felt bad about it, she was crying,' I said.

'Ah shit, I didn't mean to make her cry,' said Polly, who was finally beginning to lower her voice. She was silent. 'I guess I better apologise to her,' she said finally.

'Yeah,' I said. 'You have to be careful. It could affect your application.'

It consumed us. The Program. Polly had worked as an unaccredited registrar for a few years and was planning on applying for the Neurosurgery training program the following year. Referees were heavily weighted in the selection process. Reputation was everything.

The next day Polly apologised to the nurse. We talked about it later, and she acknowledged that she found mismanagement of neurosurgical patients triggering because of what happened to her little sister. I could completely understand. If a hospital had caused Mariko to develop a permanent neurological injury, I would be on guard too. I don't think I'd ever get over it. I really felt for Polly.

After work I caught up with Martha, whom I hadn't seen much since we'd been interns together. She was also working long hours as a resident on the surgical wards. She was currently in Urology. We'd decided to go to an evening yoga class followed by dinner. She took me to her favourite bikram yoga studio. I liked yoga because I was naturally flexible, and in a world where you're always vying for reassurance, it was comforting to definitely be good at something. Bikram yoga was intense. The room was forty degrees and humid like a tropical jungle. There was a stench of body odour which overwhelmed me. But the release I felt in that sweaty room was so addictive that the smell didn't matter.

Martha cried after the class – she said that always happened. There was something cathartic about doing a physically difficult class, which ended with a rapid breathing exercise – *kapalabhati*. Forcing yourself to breathe so quickly and climactically raised the heart rate and heightened one's emotions. And, the yoga notwithstanding, Martha was more emotional than usual that night. She had something to tell me about her boss.

'There's a thing that's started between me and one of the consultants,' she said over dinner. She told me who it was and my face fell. He was married. I felt a bit sick and didn't want to hear any more. We talked about how it had started, and I warned her as gently but as firmly as I could to stop it.

'But there's something there,' she said. 'I've told you how I've always liked older men. They're good in bed because they're experienced. They know how to treat women.'

'Treat women? Martha, he's cheating on his wife!'

'I know it looks terrible, but he says he's going to leave her,' she said.

'Please, Martha, don't get involved,' I said. 'Also, people are going to talk. They're going to think you're sleeping with him to get a good reference. Just don't do it.'

I wasn't sure if Martha was listening to me, but I couldn't believe she was even contemplating continuing with an affair that was bound to end up hurting her or this man's wife, or both of them. (Mind you, the consultant also had plenty to lose: if anyone found out he was having an affair with a resident he could be stripped of his professorship and his consultancy, as well, of course, as losing his family.) I felt fiercely morally opposed to what they were both doing. Even the next morning, I was still bothered by it, but I tried not to let it distract me. *I am a professional. I have work to do.*

I was on the ward when a paramedic wheeled in a silver-haired lady who'd been transferred from another hospital. Her name was Margot, an octogenarian with glioblastoma multiforme, the deadliest of brain tumours. Her husband,

Earle, had accompanied her in the ambulance, and we were shortly joined by their two daughters, Sheila and Alex. Once Margot was settled in her room, I took down her history and spent some time talking with her family.

'Where are you from?' they asked. *Oh, this again ...* A lot of Asian people cope with it by saying 'Melbourne'. I never bothered because inevitably the follow-up question was, 'But where are you *really* from? You know, your background?'

'I'm Japanese,' I answered.

'Oh, we love Japan. We've always wanted to take Mum to Japan to see the cherry blossoms,' said Alex.

'I've actually never seen the cherry blossoms either,' I said. 'I tend to go to Japan in summer or winter to visit my grandmother.'

We soon started talking about Japanese food, and then about cooking. I told them about the risotto recipe by Donna Hay I'd recently tried. I answered any questions they had about Margot and her admission, and finally excused myself for the evening handover meeting with the other residents, registrars and the nurse in charge of the ward.

Margot was discussed at a multidisciplinary meeting, with specialists from Pathology, Radiology, Neurosurgery, Radiation Oncology and Medical Oncology. She had a large tumour, which took up most of her brain. The consensus was that she would be a poor surgical candidate – the risks were just too high, particularly given her age and other medical comorbidities. The recommendation from the experts was that she should receive palliative radiotherapy and chemotherapy. Ultimately, the family decided they would let the disease run its course and spend the precious time left with Margot at home rather than coming in and out of hospital for treatments. I found that hard to hear, but I respected their choice. I've always wanted people to be cured, so I had this incandescent desire for patients to receive the maximum treatment possible to keep them alive. As I grew more mature, and gained more clinical experience, I realised that some patients and their families don't want that.

A few weeks later Margot passed away peacefully in the comfort of her own home, and surrounded by all of her loving family members. Her daughters came to visit me on the ward and I comforted them with cups of tea and some kind words. They brought me a card from Earle, another from them, and a couple of Donna Hay cookbooks. I was so touched. Their gestures made me understand the power of what it meant to be a doctor, just as listening to Oliver had. Sometimes it's not about saving lives or curing conditions. Sometimes it's about human connection – what we say, and how we treat patients and their families can, and does, make a difference to their experience of illness. There are fewer places where this is so starkly felt than on the Neurosurgery ward. We see such severe illnesses and injuries, it's where the power of human connection can make the most profound impact, or conversely where you can totally destroy a patient's sense of hope.

Seeing the love that Earle, Sheila and Alex had for Margot warmed me. It made me miss my own family in Sydney. I was looking forward to being with them for Christmas, my favourite time of year. I'd started buying presents for my sisters months in advance, and I couldn't wait for the big day. I always found it hard to keep secrets from them and was just busting to give them their presents.

At home, my family had decorated the top of the grand piano, draping it in a festive, poinsettia-print cloth, with a mini-Christmas tree and lots of little parcels tied with shimmering gold bows. My sisters had baked reindeer cupcakes, with red Smarties for noses and pretzels for antlers. I gave Eriko and Mariko a huge squeeze each, opened my suitcase in the middle of the living room, took out their presents and added them to the pile on the piano. Mum always asked how work was going, and I always gave a cursory reply. It was so much of an effort to try to explain the technical details of what I was doing, how the Program worked, the intricacies of my days. Besides, it was Christmas. I didn't want to bore them with medical talk.

Dad was reading a letter on the couch. He had a frown on his face.

'You're looking serious, Dad,' I said.

'It's one of my college friends,' he replied. 'He died on a plane. Heart attack.'

'Oh, that's terrible. I'm sorry.' I walked over to the couch. 'Was he a smoker?'

'No, I don't think so. They think he died from stress. He had a stressful job.'

'Wow,' I said. 'Must have been one hell of a job.'

'*Karoshi*,' he said. Death by overwork.

I wondered whether the death of his friend would change the way Hajime thought about his own work. He was a stoic man and I realised that I really had no idea whether he was currently overworked or not. That scared me. I guess I was no better. If I were stressed, I don't think I'd tell him, or Yoshiko. It was tough doing night shifts, but it was nothing to write home about.

Yoshiko walked over and gave me my Advent calendar. Eriko and Mariko had already started theirs on the first of

157

December and since it was a week before Christmas I had a lot of catching up to do. I ate up all the chocolates until that day.

'Yumiko, you're going to get the DIA-beat,' said Dad.

'Dad, I got the sweet tooth from you! Also, it's *diabetes*,' I retaliated.

'Dia-BEE-tees' he repeated, emphasising each syllable sarcastically. I chuckled and gave him one of the chocolates from my calendar.

Plastic Surgery

2013, Melbourne

From Neurosurgery, I moved on to Plastic Surgery at the start of 2013 for my surgical resident year. Like the previous year, I still had to apply, but as a doctor who'd been at the same hospital for two years, it was a little easier getting this one. A Plastic Surgery term at last! I was excited, but also apprehensive – Plastic Surgery was notorious for being the busiest term. In fact, the head of unit brought in his daughter's old bed for the registrars' office. It was fairly common for the on-call registrar to be at the hospital until the wee hours of the morning, so the bed was meant to be some sort of consolation, as if to say, *at least you don't have to sleep on the floor.*

I put a lot of pressure on myself for this term. I'd been waiting so long to be a Plastic Surgery resident. This is what I wanted to do in the future, and to have any chance of getting on to the Program, I needed to be outstanding. There were a lot of people who wanted to do Plastic Surgery. If you expressed any interest, the consultants would pretty much tell you to get in the queue. There had been three female residents in that queue last year. Charlie had already decided to enter GP training, and another girl had entered General Surgery. And then there was one. Just me.

It was a huge team. We had five registrars and three residents. My co-residents were Noah and Keith, both of whom had worked at different hospitals for their internships. I took it upon myself to lead the three of us. The registrars were also new here, having rotated through other hospitals around Melbourne in the previous year, so they were relying on me for everything from the physical shortcuts between one part of the hospital to another, to using the computer system, to knowing the people to refer to and the phone numbers for the different wards.

The Plastic Surgery unit looked after a wide range of conditions, including hand injuries and infections, complex reconstructive surgeries for major trauma and cancers, severe burns and conditions affecting the face. We had a long list of about fifty patients to see before the registrars had to go to the operating theatre, so the day started at 6.30 am.

One of the patients was Mr Scullin, whom I had looked after on Neurosurgery. He had originally been admitted to the hospital after a catastrophic bleed around his brain, an extradural haematoma. He subsequently developed a necrotic wound to his scalp – a patch of black, dead skin that would need removing and reconstructing. The Plastic Surgery team would do this using a flap of adjacent scalp that would be transposed into the necrotic part, and a skin graft. As someone who had already looked after Mr Scullin, I was invested in following him up. On the day of his surgery, I worked hard to get all of my tasks done so that I could get to the operating theatre for his operation. I was there just in time, as they were disinfecting his skin with betadine.

'Can I scrub in?' I asked enthusiastically.

'Maybe,' said Bhavesh, the senior registrar. 'Maybe not.' He passed me the betadine dish and turned his back dismissively. I held on to the dish and watched eagerly, waiting and hoping for him to turn back around to give me the green light.

'Scalpel,' Bhavesh began. 'Forceps. What's the diathermy on?'

'Thirty-five cut, thirty-five coag,' I called out, trying to help.

Bhavesh continued without acknowledging my existence. I had asked him that morning whether I could be involved in the case, so he knew I was interested, yet I felt as though I was at a party I hadn't been invited to. What did I need to do to fit in? I didn't understand. I stayed for another twenty minutes and then realised that I wasn't going to be included, so I quietly left.

'*Hey!* How was the case?' asked Noah, one of my fellow residents.

'Oh, I didn't get to scrub in.'

'What? But you were so excited about it. Why?'

'Well, I asked if I could and Bhavesh said "Maybe, maybe not" and then he ignored me after that. Maybe they're busy and thought that having to show me stuff was going to slow them down? I don't know.'

'Oh. Sorry, mate, that sucks,' he said, patting me on the back.

'Thanks, Noah. Anything on the ward I can help with?'

'Nah, it's all good. You did most of it this morning before you went down to theatre. We should go and grab a coffee before we get paged.'

'Good idea. I'll get Keith.'

The three of us went down to the café and sat there waiting for the ward to page us. In the meantime, the registrars must have finished operating on Mr Scullin because they walked past us.

'What are you bludgers doing down here? Shouldn't you be on the ward?' That was Bhavesh looking at us sharply through his rimless glasses. My heart sank. I felt like I couldn't do anything to impress him. Was I meant to feel guilty for taking a break? How audacious of us to grab coffees.

It was still early on in the term, so I remained hopeful and keen to make a good impression. Igor was the registrar on call that day. He had a reputation for being a bully at a previous hospital. Apparently one of his female interns had decided to wear pink scrubs to work one day, and he asked her, 'What the fuck are you wearing?' and made her cry. Poor girl. No one deserves to be ridiculed like that.

There were many cases to do in the operating theatre that day. Igor was operating on a hand fracture using a method called the Ishiguro technique. I felt some patriotism that in 1997 the technique was pioneered by a Japanese surgeon – it really was an elegant procedure used to fix a fracture called a bony mallet. It's a type of fracture where a fragment of bone involving the end joint of a finger gets broken off. One wire stops that fragment from displacing backwards, and another wire holds the joint in place. Igor drew me a diagram to explain it to me. Just beautiful.

Since things were piling up in the Emergency Department, I offered to clerk the patients for Igor. By working as his proxy, I took this as an opportunity to step up. I would be the one assessing the patients and coming up with a provisional diagnosis and treatment plan. I ran up and down between theatres and ED to see patients and then report back to Igor.

Before I knew it, it was already 1.30 am. I was exhausted. The long days were starting to get to me. I'd just told Igor about a patient with an injury to the tip of his finger – a nail-bed injury, which would require a small procedure. Most operations were carried out in the operating theatres, but small procedures such as the repair of a nail bed were typically done in the ED under a local anaesthetic. Unfortunately I hadn't learned how to do a repair of this kind yet. I wished that I had, so that I could've been more useful.

I went back down to ED for one last patient to see. He'd broken his hand from punching a wall. Bhavesh called these 'idiot fractures', technically known as a fifth metacarpal neck fracture. I booked in the patient to follow up with us in the outpatients' department in a few days, then walked back up to the operating theatre to let Igor know about the 'idiot' and to tell him I was going home. However, after hearing my name, I stopped just in front of the door. I stood there with the nurse in charge, Margaret, who was on the night shift.

'I can't believe she can't do a nail-bed repair. For fuck's sake. How long's she been doing this term? Can't even do a fucking nail-bed repair!' Igor laughed like a hyena.

I started to burn up inside. It was nearly two in the morning – I could have gone home hours ago with everyone else, but I had chosen to stay back to help Igor out so that he didn't come out of theatre to face an ED full of angry patients waiting to see him. Margaret looked at me with empathetic eyes and asked if I was all right. I shook my head, and left as I heard her walk in and start yelling at Igor. 'Igor! Your resident heard all of that! How could you speak about her like that? Look at the time!' I imagined Margaret pointing at the clock. *Thank you, Margaret*. Theatre in-charge nurses had a lot of power and were well respected by surgeons. She didn't need to stick up for me, but I was so grateful she had. Without her having said anything, Igor wouldn't have paused to think about his words. It can be too hard for people within the same discipline to call out bad behaviour because of the structure of hierarchy – sometimes it was easier when a nurse could stick up for a doctor, or if a doctor could stick up for a nurse.

I ran up the stairs to the residents' office, sat on the computer typing up my notes for the patients I had seen on behalf of Igor, and let the salty tears run down my face and sting my skin. My mouth was parched. I felt like I'd just swallowed sand – I realised I'd barely drunk anything since breakfast. The ward lights were turned down, patients were sleeping, there were no other doctors, and the nurses were quietly writing their notes at the nurses' station on the other end of the ward. I was so angry. I couldn't believe that I'd stayed back all these hours to help that ungrateful jerk.

'Hey, there you are!' Oh god, it was Igor. 'Can you stop typing for a sec?' I stopped but I didn't want to look at him. I didn't want him to see that I had been crying so I kept staring blankly at the screen in front of me. My eyes were doubly sore: sore from crying and sore from being awake for so long.

'Look, I'm sorry about before,' he continued. *No, you aren't*. Then somehow he turned his apology into a feedback session about how I could be a better resident. 'If you're really interested in Plastics, I want to help you, but first you gotta change a few things, you know. You can't piss off your registrars. Like, the other day, when you got up and left theatre because you didn't get to scrub in. You can't be selfish like that. You have to be a team player.'

Selfish? Since I wasn't going to be able to assist the operation, I'd left to go back to the wards to help the other residents – how was that selfish? I sat in the dilapidated old office chair with one broken wheel and wished I could spin around and walk out, but the chair was stuck.

'Thanks for your feedback,' I murmured, trying to be calm as I grabbed my bag and walked out of the office. Even when these guys were forced to apologise, they managed to turn it sour. I wished I'd told him why I'd really left the theatre that day: why *hadn't* I told him? What was wrong with me – why was this place turning me from someone who was confidently outspoken to someone who didn't feel she could be? And I was dreading my alarm: I knew that by the time I got home I would only be getting a few hours of sleep.

The next morning, one of the consultant surgeons came up to me in the operating theatre. 'Margaret mentioned how hard you worked last night,' he said. 'Good on you for seeing those referrals. You'll be a reg in no time.'

That was exactly what I needed to hear. *Thank you, Margaret*. It made me realise that there were eyes everywhere. Even if Igor had been giving me a hard time, there were enough people around who were witnessing my work ethic. Sometimes you felt like you were treading water, and other times people like Margaret threw you a buoy. Off I went to theatre to watch some surgeries. This time I even got to scrub in for a few.

Our final case for the morning was a lady who had a facial injury. Igor noticed in her past medical history that she'd had a breast augmentation. I got an icky feeling in my stomach as he peeled the patient's gown up to have a look at her implants. 'Not bad,' he said, and pulled the gown back down.

After what had happened the night before, I avoided eye contact with him but I wished I could have given him a dirty look. That poor patient was anaesthetised on the operating table. Even in the cold theatre I could feel my skin heat up. Why didn't anyone say anything? Wasn't this the kind of thing that should get reported? But no one wants to be seen as a tattle-tale.

The registrars and I went downstairs to the café at lunch-time. I was the first to get my food, so I said I'd start a table in the courtyard. After I'd been eating on my own for a while, I looked inside and saw that the registrars had started a new table. Some of them locked eyes with me and then looked away. Igor and another registrar had scoffed down their lunches already and as they walked past me they started laughing. Was I back in high school? I texted Keith and Noah to come down and join me so that I didn't look so friendless.

At home that night I wondered whether I was unlucky to be working on a team like this, or whether these were the majority of personalities in Plastic Surgery. It was hard not to feel discouraged. I'd waited so long for this term and it was not at all how I'd imagined or hoped it would be.

The only person I could think of whom I trusted enough to talk to about the Plastics mob was Mary Bloom. I still considered my former consultant from General Medicine a confidante, and she was someone whose judgement and humanity I regarded highly. It helped that I knew she also respected me, and she'd been so supportive in the past. In the absence of any mentors in surgery, I went to see her and told her about the incidents with Bhavesh and Igor.

Mary was always sympathetic. I could see she felt sorry for me, but her first question floored me. 'Why don't you do Physicians' Training?' she suggested. I actually felt quite devastated. *So, is this what happens?* I thought to myself. When someone is being given a rough time, has witnessed something gross in theatre, it becomes their responsibility to change *the entire course of their training*? But I didn't want to be rude so I simply smiled, trying to look non-committal. As much as I respected and admired Mary as a physician, perhaps she was the wrong person to talk to in this instance.

I realised, too, as I left her room, that she was friends with everyone at the hospital. She was very diplomatic, and the most non-confrontational person I knew. It seemed unlikely she would stick up for me to the plastic surgeons, her fellow consultants at the hospital. Maybe she was used to this kind of behaviour from them. So what was going on here? Was it me at fault, or these major players in the hospital? I knew I couldn't complete my Plastics term successfully without their support, their teaching, at the very least without them giving me some of their time. Did that mean I just had to put up with all the degrading treatment I'd seen?

18

I don't look the part

2013, Melbourne

'You should do ENT, it's awesome!' buzzed Frank, a senior resident. He'd become a friend of mine and, unlike us beleaguered Plastics residents, he was loving his term. Frank aspired to be an ENT surgeon, so he was thrilled to be doing this rotation. I looked at Frank and thought, *that is exactly how I should be feeling about my Plastics term.* I was now five weeks in, and things had not improved. Frank shared an office with Keith, Noah, and me so he saw how weary we were. 'Look, I'll show you how to use my nasendoscope. It's pretty cool.'

It *was* pretty cool, actually. Noah was my brave volunteer. I sprayed some anaesthetic into his nose and the back of his throat. Then I passed the thin black tube down his right nostril. When I got to the back of his nose, I turned the tube down his throat. I could see his epiglottis and vocal cords through the scope. It was amazing but rather sad that playing with a piece of ENT equipment was turning out to be the highlight of the last few weeks. This was meant to be *the* term. The one that set alight the rest of my career. Yet by now I'd semi-given up. I felt excluded from interesting operations and lamented the lack of 'team'. Instead I tried to focus on what I could do, which was to continue steadfastly working on my application for the Program. I had yet another course to attend that weekend, this time on the care of the surgically ill patient.

Where the truck are you guys?

The three of us all got the notification at the same time. It was Bhavesh. Did he think that replacing 'fuck' for 'truck' made him less boorish? Keith hurriedly replied to let him know we were in the office. We'd completely forgotten about the combined meeting with Orthopaedics – or 'Awfulpaedics' as Bhavesh called them – because we were having fun for the first time in so long. Every four weeks, this meeting took place to discuss complex fractures that required reconstruction. The orthopods looked after the broken bones and the plastic surgeons covered the large open wounds with surgical flaps. We said thanks and bye to Frank and ran down the stairs to level 2, slipping into the room sheepishly to turning heads shaming us for our tardiness. At least we could divide the shame in equal thirds, I guess.

Within a few minutes I was paged to the ward. A patient was waiting there with an infected K-wire in her hand that needed to be pulled out. She'd just had surgery a couple of weeks before to wire her broken hand back together. When I got to the ward I saw Eliza, a nurse I'd worked with in the past when I was covering the wards at night.

'Yumiko! How are you? Thanks for coming. The patient's called Tammy. She's in that room there,' she pointed.

I walked in with my equipment and introduced myself.

169

'I'll have an Aussie, thanks,' said the scrawny middle-aged woman sitting on her bed holding her injured hand. Her hair was dirty, and she stared at me with vacant eyes. I could feel the hairs on the back of my neck standing up underneath my blouse. I didn't know how to respond. It was the first time a patient had ever rejected me, let alone based on colour. I was quiet for a few seconds, wondering what to do.

'I'm here to help you, but if you'd prefer a white doctor, I'll call one. I'll be back in a moment.' I walked into the supply closet and took a few deep breaths to calm down, still shocked by what she had said. I took my phone out of my skirt pocket and stared at it. Should I text Keith? Should I ask Noah to come up to the ward? I didn't want to bother them. Maybe I should just suck it up. Eliza walked into the supply room looking for me.

'Are you okay? I just spoke to the patient about how inappropriate that was. I told her you're an amazing doctor. Will you please come back?'

'I'll be right there. I just need to grab a wire holder,' I replied.

I was still raging on the inside, but I had to remind myself that I was a professional. *I am a doctor working in the public health system and I treat everyone the same. I've treated prisoners and all sorts of crooks, and now I'll add a racist white woman to that list.*

I walked back in and reintroduced myself. 'I'm Yumiko. I'm the Plastic Surgery resident and I'm here to remove that wire from your hand because it's infected. Are you happy for me to proceed?'

'Yes, sure, but please be careful. It really bloody hurts.'

'Of course. I'm just going to clean your wound gently first, and then I'll let you know when I'm about to pull the wire, okay?'

I am fine. I am professional. I am just here to do my job. I opened up the dressing pack and poured some chlorhexidine solution into the tray. I put on some gloves, soaked the cotton balls with the solution and gently cleaned Tammy's hand. It was surprisingly small, and was trembling like a baby bird.

'Okay, Tammy, I'm going to pull the wire out. I won't lie, this can hurt sometimes, but I'll do it as quickly and gently as I can. Are you ready?' She nodded. 'All right, three, two, one . . .' and the wire was out.

'Oh, thank you. That wasn't as bad as I thought,' she said. Her forehead had tiny wet beads of anxiety strung along her wrinkles. 'And I'm sorry about before. You're great. It's just . . . I had a bad experience. There was this Chinaman in Casualty who could barely speak English and he fucked things up, you know?'

'It's okay, you don't need to explain. You're all good now. We just need to pop you back into a plaster because the wire came out a couple of weeks early. Your fracture still needs to heal.'

'Thanks, doc.'

This kind of stuff took me back to the frustrating and frankly racist comments I'd copped as an international student. And it wasn't the first time I'd heard a patient – or doctor – complain about an international medical graduate. IMGs got a bad rap: locally trained doctors considered them inferior. I didn't even know why, it's not like local doctors knew anything about medical curricula overseas. For all we knew, IMGs could have received world-class education and training. Some IMGs were still heavily accented from their place of origin, rendering them easy targets for discrimination. A lot had already finished their training overseas and were fully qualified specialists. However, if their qualifications weren't recognised in Australia, they had to retrain and start at the bottom of the food chain once more. For those IMGs, being an intern again after decades of consultant practice was bound to be demeaning. I could only sympathise. I'd hate to have to go back to the beginning.

'You know how I first broke my hand?' asked Tammy.

'No, what happened?'

'Well, I've been in this abusive relationship for seven years and we have physical fights all the time. My partner grabbed my hand and threw me against a brick wall. I passed out and I had bruises all over my face as well. See?'

I could see, and that did throw a different light on what she'd said. Not that I was excusing her prejudice, but I think people say hurtful things when they're in pain themselves.

'Yes, I can see there's still a bit of yellow around your face,' I told her. 'I presume they scanned your face when you were first seen in ED?'

'Yeah, I got the scans. All good. Anyway, I'm sorry again about before. You're a good doctor, just like the nurse said.'

'It's fine, we all say things we shouldn't say.' Suddenly I had a surge of concern for Tammy and decided that maybe I should contact the social work team. I asked her if she'd be comfortable speaking to one of them about her situation. The idea of her going back to a partner who was hurting her was terrible.

Tammy agreed, and I walked away knowing that she probably wouldn't leave her toxic relationship, but that at least I'd tried to help her. Of course, I was still hurt by her comments, but her story made me think more broadly about the experience of women subjected to domestic violence. I put the racism aside and thought about what I could do as an individual doctor. Maybe I was the first professional Tammy felt comfortable talking to about what was happening in her relationship. It was important to me that as a doctor I considered the social circumstances of a patient outside of their injury or illness.

It was a dispiriting end to my term in Plastic Surgery. Despite how I'd been treated, however, I could hold my head high. I was hard-working and resilient. I wasn't going to give up easily.

My next twelve-week term, starting in April, was supposed to be a relieving term, which meant rotating around different units and covering whomever was on leave. However, another resident didn't want to do his Neurosurgery term, and I didn't much like the idea of changing teams every week or so, so I was able to swap into Neurosurgery for round 3. I was so pleased to be back on a familiar ward with nurses whom I got along with like sisters, and with Polly. Since this was my third term with Neurosurgery I knew I'd be given a lot more responsibility. I was excited to be back, and couldn't wait to go to theatres. Anushka and the other registrars had changed around from my previous term, but Polly was still there. 'Miko!' she screamed, and gave me a giant hug. 'It's awesome to have you back on the team!'

'Thanks, Polly! So good to be back for more Nando's and Neurosurgery,' I laughed.

Sometimes I did wonder whether I would feel more included were I to pursue Neurosurgery as a specialty, or whether I was just lucky to have been teamed with Polly, as I had been unlucky to have been teamed with Igor and Bhavesh. Neurosurgery was interesting, but, despite everything, the pull toward Plastic Surgery was stronger. I maintained that Plastic Surgery was the most creative of surgical specialties and the surgeries themselves still fascinated me. Or maybe it was just out of stubbornness that I stuck to Plan A.

That morning, we admitted a new patient who had been operated on privately by a neurosurgeon called Caroline Tan. Ms Tan had put in a ventriculo-peritoneal shunt, which is a tube connecting the ventricles of the brain to the abdomen to help relieve pressure on the brain. Normally, private patients would go back to the private system, but Ms Tan was away from Melbourne. Her patient had been doing well since the operation, but he was having some mild headaches. He was admitted so we could investigate what might be wrong, and monitor him.

'Caroline? Can't look after her patients?' Prof Kaufmann scoffed and rolled his eyes when we explained the situation. 'Let's have a look at the scans.'

Polly showed Prof Kaufmann the X-rays, which showed that the shunt appeared to look fine. The CT scan of the patient's brain was unremarkable. I didn't understand where the contempt was coming from, although it wasn't unusual for Prof Kaufmann to think everyone else was inferior to him.

'Polly, what was all that about?' I asked after he'd finished the examination and left the room. 'What does Prof Kaufmann have against Ms Tan?'

'Ah . . . that,' she said, looking unsure as to how to continue. 'She took her boss to court several years ago because he showed her his dick and demanded a blow job.'

'*What?*' I said, in disbelief.

'Yeah. She won, but she's never had a job in the public system since. She's been overlooked for every job she's applied for.'

'Even though she won?'

'Yup,' said Polly and looked down. 'It's sad. The surgeons say it's because she dressed scantily and asked for it. They're such sexist pigs.'

I was so shocked I was almost speechless. Imagine studying and training for fifteen years of your life and not being able to get a job in a public hospital – the thought was devastating.

'Some neurosurgeons don't like the fact that she won. They probably feel threatened because they've been getting away with similar behaviours for so long.'

Nothing good ever comes from whistleblowing, it seemed.

Later that day I met senior registrar Cornelius, whom I knew of but hadn't worked with. He walked with a strut, parading around the ward wearing designer clothing, which was always accessorised with his favourite belt whose gigantic shiny buckle reflected the hospital lights and blinded you. He drove an expensive convertible and carried around a Gucci man-bag. I assumed from looking at Cornelius that neurosurgical registrars must earn a lot. He was the walking embodiment not only of ostentation but also of self-absorption. He was married but, I'd heard, was always cheating on his wife, like many men I'd encountered in surgery.

One night the whole team went out for drinks. By the end of the night Cornelius was making out with an orthopaedic registrar in front of all of us. I was disgusted at his blatant infidelity. Worse still, it was clear he was proud of what he saw as conquests. 'It's the five-hundred-mile rule,' he sniggered later. 'If you're five hundred miles away from your wife, it doesn't count.'

Somehow, being a senior registrar made Cornelius feel like a rock star. He had nearly finished his training and would be a fully qualified neurosurgeon soon, and that obviously gave him a sense of power. It was no surprise, then, that when a good-looking girl called Sally joined us as a reliever for a week, she was highly favoured by Cornelius. Sally was a stunning Persian woman with olive skin, brown curls and green eyes framed with long eyelashes. Even though I had been working hard on the ward, I was never picked to go to the operating theatre to assist Cornelius. I didn't look the part. That week, it was always Sally. She was happy because she didn't have to do any work on the ward, and he was happy because he got to look into her green eyes across the operating table. The favouritism was a sobering slap in the face. Just like Carlos had had it easy as a General Medicine intern, with the nurses swooning over him, Sally was cruising as Cornelius's chosen one. I hated that this was even a thing. It rocked my belief that we were in a meritocracy: it was worse than the old adage 'It's not *what* you know, it's *who* you know.' Did the men whom you worked with in this system also have to find you attractive in order for you to be able to learn from them, in order for you to advance? It was a bartering system that I didn't want to be a part of. You just couldn't win as a woman. If you weren't pretty enough, some male surgeons weren't interested in teaching you. If you were too pretty, or dressed a certain way, you were asking for sexual harassment.

19

A false farewell

2013, Melbourne

It was the middle of May, and Mother's Day fell on the same day as Mariko's birthday so I decided to head home to Sydney that weekend for the double celebration. I was allocated Thursday afternoon off, but Thursdays were busy for our team because we had Spine Clinic, which was always overbooked and consistently ran over time. I asked Cornelius if I could take Friday afternoon off instead; I figured that then I could leave a bit earlier for the airport, and it would mean more manpower for Spine Clinic. Prof Kaufmann somehow got hold of this news, and he didn't like it. The next week, he called a meeting with me and Mary Bloom. I wasn't exactly sure why Mary was asked to be there, given that she was the head of Physician Training and had nothing to do with surgery. I knew that she and Prof Kaufmann were friends so perhaps he wanted her to back him up. But I was glad she would be present.

'You know, Yumiko, you were our best resident last year,' he started. 'I don't know what happened to you but you're heading down a slippery slope.' I was shaken. Was I really getting reprimanded about an afternoon off?

'I'm sorry. I spoke to Cornelius already about my afternoon off and he approved it so I didn't think there was an issue,' I explained.

'Listen, I think you're getting too confident. This is your third term in Neurosurgery. You should know by now that as the clinical director everything has to go past me first. You think you're so important that you can take off any day you want without first asking my permission?'

'No, not at all. I asked for Friday off because it's a less busy day for the team, and I did run it by the whole team, including Cornelius.'

'But you didn't ask *me*,' he yelled, stabbing his chest with his index finger. He had a slight smile despite his aggression. It was odd, as if he were enjoying himself.

'I'm sorry. I'll ask you next time.'

'You know, I spoke to the Plastic Surgery unit about you, as well. They didn't like you. What do you think is going wrong with you?'

Prof Kaufmann knew how invested I was in Plastics. Having seen how much he promoted Neurosurgery, perhaps he was offended that I was more interested in Plastics. But . . . what *was* wrong with me? It was hard not to question myself. Surely his hectoring had nothing to do with me taking an afternoon off, which seemed inconsequential next to the darker picture he was trying to paint.

Not only were his slurs upsetting, but I was confused as to why he was taking me down. I got along with the team. I worked hard. Sure, I'd had some difficulties working with Bhavesh and Igor, but I'd forced myself to ignore their posturing, and generally I thought my rotations had been going well. Yet now I felt like I was on the edge of a precipice, about to get pushed over by him. *Just hurry up and push me already.*

Mary sat there in silence, which was unnerving. I didn't know what she was thinking. Was she taking his side? I could see that she was uncomfortable but I couldn't read her.

She did subsequently report back to the director of Medical Services that she thought Prof Kaufmann was bullying me. In the meantime, she texted me the next morning and asked to see me.

'Are you okay?' she asked with a worried look on her face. 'I couldn't sleep last night.'

'Oh Mary, I'm fine. It's okay,' I said.

'I don't think he should have said all those things to you. I know you're a good resident.'

'Thank you, I appreciate that.'

'I'm getting worried about all these bad experiences you're having in Surgery. Have you had a chance to think about physicians' training? We'll look after you,' she said. 'Please think about it, and let's meet again next week.'

I was confused. What was happening? I was so looking forward to this year. I'd finally got a Plastic Surgery rotation, and now I was back with the Neurosurgery team that I considered my 'work family'. . . except it wasn't turning out the way I'd pictured at all. The clear vision I'd had of surgery was starting to pixelate. Suddenly I'd gone from being a top dog to some rogue resident who didn't get a day's leave approved the right way. Was that really a big enough offence to dismantle me?

And now I was seriously considering the prospect of physicians' training. I didn't hate the idea of it, but it was such a mind boggle. I saw myself as a surgeon. It was part of my identity, and how people knew me. When you think 'Yumiko', you think 'surgeon'. You think of Cristina Yang from *Grey's*. Or so I hoped. Mary was right, though. Did I really want to spend the rest of my career working with people like this? How about all the courses? I'd already spent thousands of dollars of my lowly intern and resident salary on compulsory courses towards the Program. And if I chose Basic Physician Training (BPT), I'd have to give up on my application for Plastics.

I met with Mary. I decided I did need a change. Basic Physician Training. Okay. I wasn't completely comfortable with it, but I didn't see many choices. I was a little heartbroken that I'd given up. Maybe I'd succumbed to the widely held belief that women just weren't welcome in Surgery. I thought I had the balls to survive, but maybe I was too soft.

Mary explained how it would work. Since I had done a lot of Critical Care, and one Surgery term could be counted as a non-medical 'elective' term, I could go straight into the second year of BPT. That was a small consolation, that all the terms I'd already completed wouldn't go to waste.

She gave me a warm hug and I walked out of the meeting feeling both relief and remorse. Nonetheless, ever the organised type-A personality, as soon as I got home I ordered the prescribed textbook for BPT and a large tendon hammer. I had a standard tendon hammer but I was to be a BPT now so I needed the best equipment. Within a few weeks I'd completed all the assessments needed to get the first year of BPT accredited so that I could move straight into the second year.

PART 3

Registrar

20

Chicks and chooks

2013, Regional New South Wales

The menu from a Liberal Party fundraising dinner was circulating on social media in June 2013. The first dish on the menu read 'Julia Gillard Kentucky Fried Quail – Small Breasts, Huge Thighs & A Big Red Box'. I couldn't believe my eyes. How was it possible that the person holding the highest office in the country could be referred to in such an offensive, disgusting way? Even after Gillard's misogyny speech less than a year prior, there were no signs of sexism and misogyny abating in Australian politics. It also made me feel a little self-conscious as I hadn't been able to keep up my running due to the increasing workload. Not that anyone cared about my thighs.

I was heading to the countryside for the second half of 2013, for a General Surgery term. I was now in my third postgraduate year, and my rotations were a mixture of senior resident and registrar roles. These last two terms were to be registrar roles in General Surgery, and Intensive Care after that.

The change was bittersweet. On one hand, I was excited to finally be promoted to registrar level, but on the other, this was to be my last surgical rotation. Even though I had committed to doing BPT, I was still motivated to enjoy surgery and perform the best I could. I was working with a senior registrar, Mark. We shared the on-call during the week. He did Mondays and Wednesdays, and I did Tuesdays and Thursdays. We worked one in four weekends, which we shared with two other registrars from another hospital. Mark was very supportive. He knew that it was my first registrar term, so he said that I could ring him any time if I had questions I wanted to ask him before calling the boss. I was grateful for that back-up.

The roster was manageable. Sometimes I'd get the odd phone call in the middle of the night, but thankfully the hospital provided us with accommodation just ten minutes' walk from the hospital.

Surgery unknotted something in my very being. *This is fun. Am I having* fun? *Am I* allowed *to have fun?* I was cautiously jubilant. I wanted to allow myself the last hoorah, though I knew only too well by now that my joy could disappear at any time, crushed in this mortar called Surgery where anyone can act as a pestle. Nonetheless, I threw myself into the experience. I attended scope lists, and learned how to do both a gastroscopy and colonoscopy. I realise that putting tubes into orifices probably doesn't sound like fun to most of the population, but I enjoyed the technical aspects of carefully navigating around the bowel. It was trickier than expected, and that's what I loved – the challenge of a steep learning curve, and getting better and more efficient at new skills.

After a few weeks, I took my first patient to the operating theatre. It was just the incision and drainage of a skin abscess, which is not much more than popping a glorified pimple, but the responsibility made me feel like I was finally doing something worthy, something more than the run-of-the-mill discharge summaries and painkiller prescriptions, which had taken up a good part of each day previously. I was finally a registrar, not an intern or resident who takes orders from her registrars. I had my own interns, in fact. Remembering how awful the previous two terms had been, I made sure I treated my interns well. On Mondays, I asked them how their weekends were, and every morning after the ward round I would take them to the local café for a coffee and an impromptu teaching or mentoring session. At the end of each day I always thanked them for their hard work, even if they hadn't done much. It's Management 101, right? Treat your juniors well and they'll be motivated to work hard.

One day, early in my time at the hospital, I was working with Mr Grainger, a plastic surgeon to whom I'd just been explaining my 180-degree change in career direction.

'Don't you dare do Medicine,' he said as he watched me do my first rhomboid flap. 'You're a surgeon. You'd be wasted in Medicine.' We were with a patient who had a skin cancer on her face, which we were reconstructing using adjacent skin.

'You know, when most people start operating they're very tentative,' he continued, 'but not you. You take the knife and cut confidently. You don't do that thing a lot of registrars do where they take little scratches like a chook raking the ground.'

My favourite part of the term was the Plastic Surgery list because Mr Grainger let me do a lot of operating under his supervision. I did skin cancers and hand surgeries, and within a few weeks I had several cases in my logbook. It had been a while since any surgeon had taken me under their wing. I thought of Dr Stein, who had nurtured me in the last couple of years of medical school. Since then, no consultant seemed to care. I was just a worker ant in the illustrious colony of a big Melbourne hospital. Being in a smaller hospital made me feel secure. I felt more like a person than an employee.

Towards the end of term, Mr Grainger brought in some fresh eggs for me to take home. He had some chickens on his property. I opened the cardboard carton to see twelve beautiful powder-blue eggs. This was another thing I loved about rural hospitality. After I'd admired the eggs, Mr Grainger told me about an opportunity to become a plastic surgery registrar in another hospital. It was an unaccredited registrar job that would give me the experience necessary to apply for the Program; the equivalent to what Polly was doing in Neurosurgery.

Unaccredited registrar posts were hard to get in Melbourne. The hospital I was based at certainly didn't offer any to residents: in such a large and busy unit you had to have a few years of experience under your belt before you'd be considered for an unaccredited registrar job there. I couldn't quite believe this might be happening. Before going into the specifics of the job, Mr Grainger did ask me one thing, though: did I have a boyfriend? I was a little taken aback. He'd never have got away with a question like that in a formal interview setting. He explained to me that girls with partners tended to accept jobs and then pull out at the last minute because they wanted to stay with their partners. I reassured him that I was single.

'It's harder for women,' continued Mr Grainger. 'Think about it. How many female plastic surgeons do you know?'

'Hmm . . . not many. How about her?' I pointed at a photo of a female plastic surgeon on a newsletter on his desk.

'She doesn't count,' Mr Grainger said abruptly. 'She's a dyke.'

'Oh.'

'Surgery's easier when you're not going to have a kid. You're not planning on having babies, are you?' he asked.

'Not any time soon. I don't even have a man,' I laughed awkwardly.

'Good.'

It appeared I'd passed some preliminary test, but warning bells were sounding in my ears. If I were to succeed in this profession, it was obvious there were a few things I might have to keep to myself, any plans on having kids being one of them. And when was it ever acceptable to refer to a gay woman as a 'dyke', or attribute her success to her lack of children? I felt as though I was quickly learning unwritten rules I needed to follow in order to conform. I couldn't do anything about being Japanese or being a woman, but maybe there were other things I could change. I envisioned the stereotypical surgeon and my thoughts turned to the golf clubs rusting in my storage unit. I'd learned how to play golf as a teenager but it had been a while since I'd been to a driving range. Perhaps I needed to brush up on my skills. I made a mental note to bring up golf next time I had a chat with Mr Grainger.

A few weeks later, I was called for an official interview. I drove a few hours north, admiring the bright purple jacarandas against the yellow hay fields. It was the start of spring for the trees, and maybe for me, too. In a small room I was greeted by Mr Grainger, another surgeon called Mr Edgar and a lady from Medical Administration. We had what I felt was a good conversation about my experience and ambitions. Before I even got home, I received a phone call. I'd got the job. What a whiplash! Only a month or so prior I had enrolled in Basic Physician Training, and now I had been enticed back to the dark side, just like that. I told Mary straightaway. I felt guilty for quitting before I'd even begun, especially after all her support, but she understood and she was happy for me.

It was as though my brain had decided to selectively forget the abusive behaviour of surgeons over the past few years. *Surgery is beautiful.* Surgery was what I so wanted to do, and this was my ticket back into it. I was ecstatic, like I had my second wind. I would be able to start again at a new hospital, and I would once more have the chance to live up to my own expectations and become the doctor I'd always hoped to be.

21

Imposter syndrome

2013, Regional New South Wales

Mark was on annual leave, which meant I was in charge of the daily ward rounds and attended the operating lists. Day by day, I felt more grounded as a registrar, as though I was navigating the roads without a GPS. One morning I was assisting one of the general surgeons, a man called Mr Fadden. He was operating on some abdominal hernias and a few lumps and bumps. We'd spoken a few times on the phone when I was on call, but we hadn't worked with each other much. The normal small talk at the scrub sink turned into an interrogation.

'When did you graduate?' he asked.

'Two thousand and ten,' I replied. 'This is my first reg job.'

'So you're in third year?'

'Yes.'

'So you're not really a registrar, then. You're just an SRMO,' he said.

Just an SRMO. Senior resident medical officer. Ouch. Semantically, he wasn't wrong, but he'd dismissed the fact that I had been functioning as a registrar all term. I had been attending operating lists, assessing and managing patients in the Emergency, and sharing the on-call responsibilities alternately with Mark. That's not something an SRMO does. Oh well. Not all surgeons were like Mr Fadden.

The next day I worked with a lovely Japanese surgeon, Mr Nakata. Perhaps there was an unspoken bond between us as we were the only two Japanese people in the hospital in a mostly Anglo town. General surgeons in rural towns did a variety of operations, including hand surgery. Mr Nakata allowed me to operate on a man with Dupuytren's contracture, a condition in which the palm of the hand and the fingers harden and bend, causing disfigurement. This was something I never would have been able to do back in Melbourne. These cases were uncommon and complex, and there they'd have been reserved for senior registrars.

'Do you know how to do a Z-plasty?' asked Mr Nakata.

I was so glad that Mr Grainger had shown me the technique and I could reply 'Yes'.

'Go on then, draw it out,' he said, handing me over a marker. I drew the Z-plasty incision on the patient's skin by marking small oblique lines coming off the main incision.

'Very good,' he said. 'I'll watch; you continue.'

And so that day I did my first operation on a patient with Dupuytren's contracture, being very careful to dissect around the small nerves of each finger. As I tied my final knot, Mr Nakata inspected the wound. 'It looks like a plastic surgeon's been here,' he said. I couldn't have been happier in that moment. Mr Nakata's avuncular warmth was exactly what I needed after the interaction I'd had with Mr Fadden the day before. I did, however, wonder whether Mr Nakata only gave me the opportunity because I was also Japanese.

Fergus was the first reliever we had covering for Mark. Fergus had gingery-brown curls, freckles, broad shoulders and no neck. Within moments of meeting him he launched into some heavy-duty name-dropping. He was writing a textbook chapter with a famous plastic surgeon in Melbourne, and proceeded to mansplain to me the entire contents of said chapter.

'So, I'm presuming you're Japanese,' he said. '*Konnichiwa. Chotto nihongo hanasemasu*,' he continued proudly before I could answer. 'Hello. I can speak a little bit of Japanese.'

I hated when people talked at me in Japanese. It was as ridiculous as barking at a dog or cooing at a pigeon. I speak English. What made him assume that I could speak Japanese anyway?

'My last girlfriend was Asian,' he went on. 'Actually, all of my girlfriends have been Asian.'

I drank my coffee as quickly as possible. 'I might head back to the hospital. I have a few things I have to do. You take your time, Fergus.'

'Oh, I'll walk back with you,' he said.

'No, no, it's fine. I can walk by myself. You enjoy your coffee,' I said and hurried out.

Thankfully, Fergus was only around for a week. Our next reliever was Christian, who was tall and quiet. He had dark brown hair, blue eyes and big muscles. On his first day, we were paged to the Emergency Department to see a patient with a wound on his back. Christian didn't need to say a thing when we arrived.

'Hi, I'm Annalise. Let me know if you need anything,' offered a young nurse, batting her lash extensions at him and following closely behind as he went to see the patient.

'Could I have a dressing pack?' he asked.

'Oh yes, of course,' Annalise replied, and rushed immediately to get him a trolley set up with a dressing pack, cleaning solution and a selection of dressings. 'I didn't know what you needed so I brought you everything – gauze, Opsite, Hypafix . . . We have more dressings if there's something else you want?'

Later that day, we got another page about a similar patient. It was a simple abscess so I told Christian that I was fine to go on my own. I saw Annalise again, so I asked her for the same dressing set-up.

'Go to the back of the Emergency Department – you'll find the supplies there,' she said, her expression unrecognisable from the bubbly nurse who had fussed over Christian just a few hours before. Of course, this was nothing new to me: I thought back to Carlos on the General Medicine ward in Melbourne, and his effect on the nurses there. Male doctors, it seemed, just needed to be confident. Handsome male doctors just needed to be handsome. Women doctors just needed, apparently, to wear pearls and a chignon, and spend weeks engaging in girly chats with the female nurses to gain their support.

After my term as a rural general surgery registrar I was seconded to a small Melbourne hospital for Intensive Care. There was an arrangement made that my base hospital would send a few of their doctors to the smaller one, and vice versa. Kind of like an exchange program. Mr Grainger, however, had other ideas. I received a phone call from him not long after I was back in Melbourne. His rural unit was going to be under-staffed and he asked me to break my contract and come to work for him earlier than agreed, before I'd finished in Melbourne. He wasn't taking no for an answer.

'Do you want to do ICU or do you want to become a plastic surgeon?' he asked. Even down the phone I could feel the pressure he was piling on. He knew that would be the perfect emotional bargaining tool.

'A plastic surgeon,' I replied immediately.

'So? The answer should be easy.'

'I know, but I'm contracted until the end of the year. I can't break a contract.'

'Why not?'

I paused. I didn't know how to answer. 'Well,' I continued, 'it's frowned upon to break a contract. I'd have to be replaced for the last two weeks. I don't think it would be fair to my department.'

'We can offer you locum rates,' he said to entice me.

'I really don't think I should break the contract,' I said one more time.

'You think about what you want for your future,' he said as he hung up. Still holding the phone to my ear, I felt very uncomfortable as the tone reverberated. He was making me do the wrong thing, but I don't think he cared. All he cared about was ensuring his unit was staffed.

The next day, a lady from Medical Administration rang, having put together a contract that showed no intention of paying me locum rates. The phone rang again moments later. It was Mr Grainger.

'So, you're coming, aren't you?' Mr Grainger's voice echoed down the line.

'Yes. Yes, okay,' I replied, overwhelmed. I succumbed to his pressure, reluctantly broke contract and started two weeks early at my new job. The whole thing made me very uneasy, not least because I was worried I'd be blacklisted by Melbourne. Nevertheless, almost without meaning to, I dropped my life there and moved.

My new hospital had a team of four registrars and a rotating roster of consultants who visited from Sydney or Melbourne a week at a time – we didn't have any consultants who were full-time. The senior registrar was Lars, an international medical graduate. He had been at the hospital for a number of years. The other three of us were new. Trevor was a short Welshman. Nina was a lovely, introverted woman from England, who was new to Plastic Surgery. She had been working in Emergency as a resident but was interested in surgery. For the first time in my life I was the 'Aussie' of the group, which felt odd indeed. Having arrived here at the age of fifteen, I had developed an Australian accent with only a hint of English from my time in London, and a slight Japanese twang.

I was a newly minted plastic surgery registrar. When I was on call, I was the 'expert' on all things Plastics.

Except I wasn't. I still didn't know enough to be confident of giving advice. I felt like an imposter. Between internship and now, my confidence levels had dropped: it was hard to maintain any self-belief after some of the things that were said to me in Melbourne by the likes of Prof Kaufmann, Igor and Bhavesh.

About a week into the new job I was feeling so out of my depth that one day after work I started to tear up in the car park. I rang Martha from my car. Being the superstar that she was, she had got on to the Program for General Surgery, and had just started her first term as an accredited registrar.

'I don't know what I'm doing. I'm a total fraud,' I lamented. 'I don't have any friends here, and I miss Melbourne.'

22

Euro-vision

2014, *Regional New South Wales*

Over the next few weeks, I felt less like an imposter. I knew I could give simple advice over the phone, and I was finding comfort in my routine. Ward rounds started at 7 every morning, but I wanted to keep up my fitness so I joined the gym down the road from the hospital, which opened at 5.30. I timed everything to the minute. I woke up every morning at 5. I gave myself fifteen minutes to get ready, and drove ten minutes to the gym, arriving five minutes before the doors opened. Once I was there, I exercised for an hour until 6.30, showered, left the gym by 6.45, and was on the ward by 7. The military precision was, I discovered, absolutely essential for my mind. In an unpredictable world like the hospital, this morning routine gave me a sense of order – it centred me. You never know what might come through the Emergency doors, or how late you'll have to stay back each day.

The gym also gave me a sense of community outside the hospital. I became friends with Cara, one of the trainers there.

Through Cara I became friends with May, an Australian-born Chinese woman. May was a great friend who was very sympathetic towards my schedule. She lived close to the hospital, and on days when I finished work late she'd offer to cook dinner and have a hot plate waiting for me when I got there. It was like I had my own wife, something a lot of professional women envy about their straight male colleagues who have wives pandering to their needs. Certainly that was the case for Lars and Trevor, who had wives at home to cook and clean after them.

I quickly learned on the job and by March I was in my stride. Apart from Nina, who was a single woman in her late twenties like me, the other registrars enjoyed married life, and Lars had a daughter, so we were at different life stages and didn't have much in common. While I prioritised things like getting my endorphin fix through exercise, their spare time was spent with their families. It wasn't the same as working with the likes of Polly, Anushka, or Charlie, but they were nice enough. In any case, I was too focused on strengthening my Program application for Plastic Surgery to make new friends. I needed to have more research on my CV. Mr Grainger was interested in reconstructing hand injuries using a specialised method he'd been refining over recent years. I put together a case series of the relevant operations he had performed, which I thought I could present at two European conferences later in the year. I summarised the study in an abstract – a shortened, digestible version – and submitted it to each of the conferences.

Around that time, I remember a turning point clearly. We had a lot of operations to do one afternoon and I was given the 'easy' case as the junior registrar.

'It's a superficial cut on the forearm – just stitch it up. That's all you have to do,' said Lars.

That sounded okay. I proceeded to my allocated operating theatre.

Sophia, the head nurse for Plastics, was there getting things ready. She was always very organised and efficient. I said hello and checked that we had all the equipment I would need. I felt calm. Hand surgery was becoming a routine now. Prep. Drape. Squeeze the forearm and hand. Turn up the tourniquet up to 250 mmHg. Off we go.

'Happy for me to start?' I asked the anaesthetist. I got the nod of approval.

I followed first principles. I opened up the wound. It was not 'just' a cut. The wound went deeper, so I explored the injury carefully. Already I saw a nerve and a tendon that had been transected. My heart was racing, but on the exterior I tried to look relaxed.

'It's not just a laceration. This case will take a bit longer, sorry,' I informed the anaesthetist and nurses. 'I need to repair a nerve and a tendon.'

I opened up the wound so that I could see the extent of the injury better. I knew what I had to do. By the time the consultant, Mr Edgar, walked into the theatre, I had already finished repairing the nerve and tendon. He looked over my shoulder. 'Tell me what you've done,' he said.

'I've just repaired the SRN and FCR,' I replied, pointing out the nerve and tendon with my forceps. My heart rate went up a little as Mr Edgar scrutinised my work. Suddenly the stitches I'd made felt like they were being projected onto a movie screen.

'Good,' he said, and walked out again.

I sighed with relief.

'Saline wash, please. I'm closing,' I announced. Inside, I felt triumph rise in my chest, like the glorious morning sun. I'd just finished my first exploration of a forearm wound.

That was the day I knew that I would be able to handle anything thrown my way. *Just stick to first principles*, I told myself.

I vividly remember walking to the staff car park. The sweet sunset was striated marmalade and strawberry. I called Martha. On the General Surgery program she was experiencing a lot of 'firsts' too – I knew she'd understand my excitement. However, it turned out that Martha had other problems. She had been seeing that surgery professor for two years now, and she was completely distraught because she was in love and he hadn't left his wife yet.

'What?' I was shocked and confused. 'Hold on. Two years? So, you mean when you first told me about him you were already serious?'

'Yes,' she admitted.

'Oh, Martha . . . I told you not to go there.' I felt ill.

'I know, but it was too late.'

'Jesus . . . I thought you had only dipped your toes in the water.'

'Nope, I dived right in and now I'm drowning,' she said. 'He keeps saying he'll leave his wife but it's been two years and he still hasn't. I don't know if I can keep doing this.'

'Martha, I don't think they ever do leave,' I said. 'He's an eminent professor with a family. Do you think he's going to disassemble that perfect picture? It will completely ruin his reputation.'

'No, I guess not,' she said. 'But I don't know what to do.'

I told Martha again that she needed to leave immediately. She was already on the General Surgery training program and needed to study for her first exam, the surgical primaries: a barrier exam usually taken in the first year of the Program, which tested Anatomy, Physiology and Pathology. It was an exam that unaccredited registrars could take, too, and its results would count towards the Program application, so it was on my mind. This year I was focused on gaining operative experience in hand surgery, and completing research projects, so I'd decided that next year would be the right time for me to enrol for the surgical primary exam. I was constantly checking off things I'd done for my CV, and adding those that still needed to be done, as though working on a rotating mood board. Martha had already ticked all of these things, and I didn't want her to waste her hard-earned position by getting entangled in this extra-marital mess. I was rooting for her to ace these exams. We were meant to be surgical buddies, like Cristina Yang and Meredith Grey. We needed to do this, together.

Building on the confidence from the day before, I was forced to step up again when a woman came in with an amputated finger. My heart was pounding hard against my ribs as my feet pounded the corridor towards the Emergency Department – it was time-critical. An amputated finger was one of the few true surgical emergencies in Plastics. In a cubicle I found Rhonda, a woman in her forties clutching a plastic bag with her finger in it. She'd been using a circular saw at home, which had gone completely through her left index finger.

For someone who had just chopped off her finger, Rhonda was remarkably calm. After assessing her, I called Mr Edgar, who was the surgeon on call. Theoretically, I knew that this finger should not be reattached. It had been amputated at the base of the finger, and in those cases, a replant means the patient ends up with a stiff, numb finger. It's essentially like having a wooden stick rather than a functional finger, so it's more of a nuisance; a patient such as Rhonda often comes back months down the track to have the finger removed.

I knew I had to be honest with Rhonda and give her all the information, but it felt awkward to present my professional opinion: that we wouldn't normally bother reattaching it. Rhonda insisted that she wanted her finger put back on, and I could empathise with that. I don't know how I'd feel with a body part missing either. This was a difficult dilemma. I relayed this information to Mr Edgar, who made the ultimate call. We would be reattaching the finger.

I galloped up the stairs to the operating theatre to book Rhonda's case. I emphasised the urgency of the operation and started mobilising the team, ensuring we had the microscope and all other equipment ready. My adrenaline levels were high. It was my first time to assist in microsurgery, and I was excited, although still a bit uneasy about the decision, knowing that Rhonda may not get a good outcome. I wondered whether the wooden-like appendage on her hand would indeed eventually annoy her later on, once all the wounds had healed.

Trevor had a problem with me assisting Mr Edgar. Technically, the registrar who was on call the day before – Lars in this instance – was allocated to emergency theatre, but I was on call and would be taking over from 5 pm anyhow. So, for continuity of care it made sense for me to be there from start to finish instead of playing tag-team with Lars. Microsurgery was intense, and changing over in the middle of it would be disruptive. I think there was perhaps a bit of competitiveness getting in the way because we all wanted to be involved. This was the first replant surgery we'd had at this hospital, and possibly the last, given how uncommon they were. Out of respect, I spoke to Lars about it, and he was fine with me doing the operation. Trevor was most displeased.

After that short sideline, I got Rhonda ready for surgery. There was a lot of nervous energy in the room. I knew this was a big moment. Mr Edgar's voice boomed down the corridor, accompanied by the percussion of his wooden clogs. He had arrived. We sat opposite each other and worked under the microscope. It really tested my hand–eye coordination in a new way. I think maybe Dad teaching me how to touch-type as a kid helped, although this of course was much harder. My eyes faced forward to look down the eye pieces of the microscope, at the image of my hands, which were just about waist level. It was a strange sensation to not be looking directly at my hands moving, as if I was disconnected from them. A few hours passed, and Mr Edgar was getting increasingly frustrated. It wasn't going well and I didn't know how to make it better. I was finding it hard to move the blood vessels exactly how he wanted me to.

'You're useless!' he screamed. 'I may as well be operating on my own, you're not helping!'

I looked at the clock. Midnight. My eyes started to well up as Mr Edgar continued to berate me. He was struggling to get the blood vessels together, and I felt jammed. It was like driving a car with a passenger saying 'Go there! There! No, there!' Go where? We got nowhere.

The surgery ended up taking twelve hours. We did eventually get there. Afterwards, I stayed awake for a while. I was upset about getting yelled at, and about Trevor guilting me for operating instead of Lars. I wrote an email to the other registrars about what we should do next time this sort of thing happened. I was firm in my belief that the patient always comes first, and that we as a team should take the course of action that best allowed for continuity of care.

Later that day, I went to talk to Mr Grainger about some research topics. When I got to his office, he informed me of a complaint. Trevor had reported me for the email I sent last night. I was shocked. Couldn't Trevor have talked to me himself?

'Look,' Mr Grainger said. 'You can't trust this guy. Don't write any more emails.'

'Okay,' I replied. 'I'm sorry. I just really felt strongly about defending my position.'

I was relieved that Mr Grainger was on my side even though Trevor had tried to undermine me. We moved on to discuss research. Having submitted my abstracts to the European conferences, I was itching to start a new project. I spoke to Mr Grainger about a few topics, and we decided upon osteoarthritis of the thumb. There were several surgeries to treat this painful condition, and one of the more novel approaches was to sever the nerves that supply the joint. I worked with Mr Grainger to develop a questionnaire to ask patients before and after their procedure to see whether this surgery made a difference to their pain and hand function.

As the weeks went by, I discovered a passion for hand surgery. Plastic Surgery was a very diverse specialty – surgeons literally operated from head to toe – and hand surgery was slowly forming a special place in my heart. Operations to treat carpal tunnel syndrome and trigger finger were relatively simple, but satisfying because they made such a difference to patients' lives. Patients with severe carpal tunnel syndrome lost sleep because the pins and needles in their hand would wake them up at night. They had trouble doing everyday things such as carrying the groceries. The surgery to treat the condition took just ten minutes, and patients would feel immediate relief – small action, big impact. Hand surgery was wonderful like that.

With four registrars sharing the on-call roster, it was manageable. Even if your twenty-four hours on call were busy, you had a few nights off afterwards to catch up on sleep.

One night I was woken up at 3 am by a doctor calling to book a patient into the fracture clinic. I thought every doctor knew that you don't call someone in the middle of the night unless you really have no choice. A clinic appointment was far from an emergency. I was cross as I tried to get back to sleep. At 3 you're in the middle of deep sleep, you get startled by the ring tone, and you have to wake yourself up to give advice over the phone. Once you're fully awake it's hard to fall asleep again: you often think about the conversation after you've finished, replaying it in your head to make sure that you gave the right advice. You hardly ever feel refreshed the next morning after a call at that time of night. It made me think about all the sleepless nights Polly and Anushka used to talk about. They would've been rung for things like catastrophic brain bleeds, though. I'm not sure they ever took appointment bookings in the dead of the night. Or did they?

Sure enough, I felt groggy the next morning as I walked to the operating theatre. That day we had a medical rep there during a complex hand surgery. She was from a medical device company that made the plates and screws we were using. Trevor was being weirdly friendly towards her – he complimented her skin, her necklace, her watch, her shoes. Anything he could see.

'I asked the rep to give us spots in a hand fracture workshop her company's running,' Trevor told me after she'd gone.

'Oh wow, that's amazing. I thought they were only for advanced trainees?'

'Yes, but I convinced her to let us go,' he said. 'But I need to send her the application tonight. Can you email your CV to me?'

'Yes, of course. Thanks so much,' I said. He knew I had a great interest in hand fractures, but I was surprised he'd included me in this opportunity. Perhaps he was extending an olive branch after throwing me under the bus to Mr Grainger. I really wanted to go to this fracture workshop, so even though I wasn't totally comfortable doing it, after a bit of hesitation, I emailed him my CV that afternoon. CVs were not usually shared around, particularly among registrars who were not yet on the Program. Selection was so highly competitive that candidates kept their accomplishments to themselves, a bit like playing poker. Once you were considered a threat, it changed how people treated you.

It turned out I should have listened to my gut, because the fracture workshop Trevor was supposed to have applied for on my behalf never happened. I wondered if he'd made the whole thing up, in fact. I confided in Nina about the incident and she wasn't surprised. 'You're both competing for the Program at the same time,' she said. I guess Trevor didn't think Nina was a threat because she wasn't planning on applying any time soon as she was a couple of years younger than us and wasn't even sure if she wanted to do Plastics in the long run. On the other hand, Trevor and I were at the same stage of our careers. And I should have known that he wasn't the type to help out a direct competitor. Not only that, but it turned out he had been attending a Cleft Clinic at the hospital without the rest of the registrars knowing. The surgeons at this hospital did not operate on children with cleft lip and palate deformities, so surgeons visiting from interstate ran a clinic every few weeks instead. One, a highly regarded doctor, was involved in the selection and education of Plastic Surgery trainees. A very important contact for Trevor. Despite my growing interest in hands, I would have loved to learn about cleft lip and palate surgery, too. It was an area of Plastic Surgery I'd had little exposure to, and I was always hungry for more knowledge and experience. But this opportunity was firmly closed to me now: Trevor had already asked Mr Grainger for Fridays off whenever the Cleft Clinic was scheduled, and we were never allowed to have more than one person off work, otherwise we would be understaffed.

23

If you are the one

2014, Regional New South Wales

A text message arrived from Mr Grainger on a Friday afternoon. 'Call me tomorrow, mid-morning.'

The next day at around 10 am I called him.

'I said mid-morning,' he growled, without saying hello first.

'Oh, I'm sorry, I thought ten o'clock was mid-morning,' I replied, a little surprised. Surgeons start the day early, so I thought ten might even be considered late morning.

'It's fine,' he sighed. 'You're going to Europe, congratulations.'

'Europe? So our abstract got accepted?'

'Oral presentation.'

'Wow, this is amazing!' I couldn't believe it. I hadn't been to many conferences before, let alone one in Europe, let alone at the Plastic Surgery Congress, which only happened every four years. It felt like I was going to the Olympics.

There were 'oral' and 'poster' presentations at medical conferences. For poster presentations, candidates printed their research onto a large poster for an exhibition. Oral presentations meant that you got to give a talk to an auditorium of surgeons. I would have been happy enough with a poster presentation, but getting to *speak* at the conference was beyond my wildest dreams. I was both nervous and excited. Nervous, because the crowd would be filled with consultant plastic surgeons from all over Europe, but excited for the incredible opportunity.

As soon as I got off the phone from Mr Grainger, I called my parents. I could tell from their voices that they were impressed and happy for me. We hadn't been back to Europe since we'd lived in London all those years ago. I was filled with nostalgia as we spoke about our lives back then. My parents passed the phone to Mariko, who was starting her fourth year of Commerce/Law at the University of Sydney. At that stage she was unsure whether she would follow in Eriko's footsteps to become a lawyer, although I'm sure she would've felt compelled to. None of us had been coerced into our areas of study, but I often wondered if we truly did choose Medicine and Law ourselves, or were we subconsciously manipulated into the model minority myth? It was hard to know whether any of us had dismissed other interests or degrees because they didn't fit into the Asian stereotypes that are so tightly woven into the fabric of society. I told Mariko that a Law degree would open many doors, and she needn't feel pressured. It was somewhat different to Medicine, which was a vocational degree. When you study Medicine, you become a doctor. There's no deviation from the factory line.

After talking to my family, I called Martha. She had been so preoccupied by her issues with the professor that she had failed her primary surgical exams. *This is why it's better not to have a man in your life*, I thought. *It's too much of a distraction*. I then spoke to Polly, who was also having some boy issues. She was seeing a man who wasn't interested in committing. She too had failed her exams recently. What was going on? I hated that both of these talented women could be derailed by their relationships. I was glad that I was relatively problem-free and had a trip to Europe to look forward to, which I would take on my own to do what I wanted. I didn't need to make sure that my partner could get leave at the same time, or have to put together an itinerary that we both enjoyed. It was something just for me.

Back at work on Monday, I couldn't stop smiling. Mr Grainger was proud of me and had already told the team, though I wished he hadn't, because I didn't want to give Trevor something to resent me for, given how ruthlessly competitive he was.

After work May invited me over to celebrate. It was nearly winter, so the hotpot she prepared was a treat. Cara brought over some drinks and we turned on the telly to watch the latest episode of *If You Are the One*, a Chinese dating show. A gorgeous twenty-eight-year-old woman was a contestant on the show. Even though I was reading subtitles, she came across intelligently in the way she communicated. She was a highly successful businesswoman in China and referred to herself as a *sheng nu*.

'What's a *sheng nu*?' I asked May.

'Oh, it means "leftover woman",' she explained.

'Left over? What does that even mean?'

211

'In China, any woman who's twenty-seven and still unmarried is called a "leftover".'

'That's so horrible! We're going to be leftovers soon,' I said, realising that I was turning twenty-seven in a few months.

My abstract on hand reconstruction was also accepted for the second European conference I'd applied to. My heart was jumping up and down like a kid on a pogo stick. Europe just got a little bit hotter! I was glad to be leaving winter to head to Lyon first, to present a poster, and then Barcelona for my oral presentation a couple of weeks after that. The news put me in a good mood for the operating list that afternoon and I had a theatre to myself so I got to put on my own playlist. I made sure to include Cyndi Lauper's 'Girls Just Want to Have Fun'. We had an all-female team that day – the anaesthetist, anaesthetic nurse, scrub nurse and scout nurse were all female – so I played all my girly tunes from the eighties and nineties.

'What the hell is this? I feel like I've just walked into a tampon commercial!' yelled Mr Edgar as he strode into the theatre.

'Good afternoon, Mr Edgar.'

'Good afternoon, Dr Kadota. What are you doing in here?'

'I'm doing the hand traumas. About to do a bony mallet.'

'Excellent, very good, I'll leave you to it,' he said. I could hear the click-clack of his wooden clogs as he entered the next-door operating theatre where Trevor was. The consultants got paid a fee-per-service, so on days when the registrars each had an operating theatre, they really hit the jackpot. On Fridays, when Mr Edgar was running a clinic, he'd gallop chaotically between the outpatient department on the ground floor and the operating theatres on the first, collecting patient labels and making sure that his name was on the attendance sheet so that he could claim a fee. There was even one case at which he managed to arrive after I'd already put the dressings on. He added an extra piece of tape to secure the dressing, and signed off his name. Imagine getting paid thousands of dollars just to put a Band-Aid on a finger.

I still had residual memories of Igor first teaching me about bony mallet fractures when I was a resident. It didn't take anything away from the surgery, though. The Ishiguro technique had become my favourite procedure. I always found it to be an elegant approach, and I never got bored of it. Another bony mallet procedure was under my belt. I ripped my disposable scrubs off with great satisfaction as I went to write up the operation report.

'Three minutes, K-wire queen,' called Sophia from outside the theatre. She had been timing me. 'Not bad, not bad,' she said with a proud look on her face. I smiled back. Sophia liked fast operators.

A few weeks later it was finally time for my big European adventure. My first stop was Lyon via Paris to visit my friend Esther, who was in my Year 12 maths class and now living over there. I stayed in Porte de Champerret, in the seventeenth arrondissement. Even though I was in France, I really wanted a good old Australian flat white, and Esther knew just the place. I didn't want to take the Metro, I wanted to explore Paris by foot, so I embarked on a big walk to meet her. It was a warm and gorgeous Parisian summer's day – perfect. I strolled down the famous Avenue des Champs-Elysées, crossed the sparkling River Seine over Pont Alexandre III, and then passed the museum of Rodin to my left and the tomb of Napoleon to my right. Ah, Paris, the most beautiful city in the world. Esther took me to a café partly owned by an Australian man. Seeing 'flat white' on the otherwise French menu filled me with sweet delight. I felt like such an Aussie in that moment. I had lived in Australia for over a decade by then, and I had really developed a fondness for my adopted country.

After a few days in Paris, I took the rail to Lyon. Walking into the conference venue, I saw my poster projected on a large screen in the foyer, and surgeons walking by, reading all the posters. It was an exciting time.

The conference in Barcelona was equally charming. I wasn't sure when I would next be able to go on such a trip, so I savoured every moment of my first day there, regaled by the striking architecture of Gaudí and the delightful food of Catalonia.

My presentation was the following morning. I walked into a large auditorium with velvet seats filled with surgeons from all over Europe and found my seat. I could feel my heartbeat get faster as my turn to speak approached; I began gripping the programme so tightly that it was getting creased and a little sweaty in my hand. My eyes kept bouncing between it and my watch, counting down the minutes before it was time for my presentation.

When it was finally my turn, I caught words in different languages waft in and out from each row as I walked down the steps towards the stage. After a little stumble with the laser pointer, which I couldn't get to turn on, I started. I spoke lucidly for my allocated ten minutes, and fortunately for me the audience didn't have any hairy questions.

Afterwards, Mario, an Italian plastic surgeon, came up to me to chat further about my talk. It felt surreal. A fully qualified surgeon talking to *me*? He wanted to discuss the technique that his unit was using for the same flap I described, as they were doing things slightly differently in Italy. I thanked Mario for sharing his expertise. Since I myself would not be performing the complex procedure, I passed on his words to Mr Grainger.

Back in Australia in July, Mr Grainger was trying to recruit a replacement for Nina, whose contract was ending – she was heading back to the UK. Even though her contract was always going to expire halfway through the year, Mr Grainger was furious. 'There's no point in training her if she's leaving,' he told the rest of us. 'Just keep her in the clinic, don't let her go to the operating theatre. She's disloyal.'

'Yes, of course,' replied Trevor. Lars and I looked at each other and didn't say anything. I was guilt-ridden. It was unfair. All junior doctors deserved to be trained. I knew I should defend Nina, but I honestly couldn't bear the prospect of facing Mr Grainger's vitriol. I still had six more months at this hospital. I knew that if I disagreed with him, he would give me a hard time and call me disloyal too.

That morning, I was assigned to run the clinic. I was seeing an elderly male patient who had injured his thumb on his farm and I could tell that he wasn't looking after himself. His sun-tanned skin was flaky like a croissant. I remembered how much the elderly patients had loved getting their hands moisturised when I'd worked as an aged care volunteer as a medical student, so I decided I'd offer him the same treatment. It was a quiet day, so I had the time to give that extra TLC. I picked at the flakes and then rubbed the moisturiser gently on his hands. 'That feels lovely, dear,' he said. I smiled back.

As the patient was leaving the clinic, a red-faced Nina walked in on the verge of tears. I asked her what was wrong; I had never seen her so upset before.

'Mr Edgar's sent me to swap with you,' she said.

'But you're assigned to theatres today,' I said. 'Was it an operation you couldn't do?'

'No, it's a nail-bed repair. I can do those,' said Nina. 'He said to get you to do it.'

Mr Edgar was obviously another one obeying captain's orders. I couldn't believe how rancorous Mr Grainger was, and that Mr Edgar, who was a consultant colleague, not a junior as we were, was a willing accomplice.

The incident made me want to leave this place even more. I was already planning on applying to Sydney hospitals for the following year because there was a better chance of getting on to the Program from Sydney. The selectors for New South Wales all worked there, so there was no point in staying where I was. I felt that I had learned what I needed to learn here, and another year wouldn't add much to my clinical experience. It was common practice for registrars to move every year to make new contacts and broaden their experiences, as each hospital had a different case mix. After spending four years away from home, I was looking forward to being near my family again, too.

In August, I applied for Plastic Surgery unaccredited registrar jobs in Sydney and was given an interview at a hospital in Western Sydney. Initially, Trevor failed to get any interviews in Sydney. He didn't look particularly impressed that I had one. After making a phone call, however, he somehow had interviews for all the hospitals in Sydney by the afternoon. How was that even possible? I later found out he'd spoken to the cleft palate surgeon he knew, who happened to be closely linked to the job selection in Sydney.

I told Mr Grainger that I was applying for jobs in Sydney, and later that week he organised a one-on-one mentoring session at a steakhouse. He asked for his steak well done – 'As black as your dress,' he said as his eyes ran down the waitress's body and back up again.

Once our food arrived, his sinewy fingers grabbed a knife and fork, cutting his black steak into evenly-sized tiny squares. He tried to convince me to stay working with him. I had planned to tell him as diplomatically as I could that I felt there were limited career prospects where I was, but in the end he became so aggrieved at the idea of my leaving that I didn't bother. Instead I said I was missing my family too much, which was not untrue.

Even then the conversation turned sour. 'If you leave, I'll have to give the research project to one of the new registrars coming to the unit next year,' he said. I took a gulp of my water and nodded in silent resignation. I had spent all year collecting the data for my study on osteoarthritis of the thumb, but as my supervisor for the project, Mr Grainger had the power to take it off me and get someone else to continue. Yet, even though I was about to lose this publication opportunity, I knew

I couldn't stay. I would never get on to the Program if I didn't move to a bigger hospital in Sydney.

Trevor and I both secured jobs in Sydney. He got his first choice, working with the surgeon from the cleft clinic, and I was given the job in Western Sydney. As the hospital was located a long way from my family, I planned on finding an apartment between there and the CBD so I could still be within reasonable distance of them.

Mr Grainger was furious. He cancelled Christmas. Each year, every unit of the hospital held Christmas parties for their registrars, but this year the Plastic and Reconstructive Surgery Unit had no such event.

After I left I received an email from the unit secretary. It was a formal letter advising me not to publish any of the data I had collected for my research project. Goodbye to you, too, Mr Grainger.

24

Fucking hand surgeries

2015, Sydney

The daily commute to the hospital was a straight line along the motorway. There was something comforting about the monotony of following a flat grey road for forty minutes. It was the only time of day that I could just sit still and not think about anything. My brain was in autopilot, my car was in cruise-control, and the only thing moving was my hand adjusting the steering wheel to stay in my lane.

From my first week at my new hospital, I was entrusted to do a lot of things on my own. On the team was Jack, a Plastics registrar, and two other unaccredited registrars, Asif and Rasheed, who were IMGs – Asif from Iraq and Rasheed from Bangladesh. Jack was often with the consultant surgeons in their operating rooms, while the rest of us took turns operating on trauma patients coming in with hand and facial injuries. Jack was in his third year of the Program, which meant he got a lot of one-on-one time with the consultants so they could teach him how to do the more complex operations.

We also had three outpatient clinics a week to follow up the patients we'd operated on. On Mondays the Plastics clinic ran concurrently with the ENT one. I became friends with Jisoo, an unaccredited ENT registrar who used a consulting room next to mine. Apparently it was confusing for the nurses in the clinic because she and I were the only two Asian female surgical registrars in the hospital. I kept getting called 'Jisoo', and vice versa. Jisoo was Korean. I was Japanese. We looked nothing like each other except that we both wore glasses. We laughed it off, but it did get annoying after a while.

Jisoo was applying for the ENT training program that year. We talked about how competitive the process was, and we both decided that this year we should sit the surgical primary exams, which were in October. They weren't early enough to count towards this year's application, but they would count towards next year's. It was very rare for doctors to be accepted on to the Program on their first attempt . . . unless you're Anushka. Everyone else I knew had taken a few tries. But just say we were successful on our first go, taking the exams would still be beneficial because we'd have to take the same ones in our first year of training anyway.

I drew up a schedule to ensure that we would cover all topics by October. Jisoo and I started meeting up every week to study.

I was on call on Monday 9 March. I was in the operating theatre in between cases when a nervous intern called me about an elderly man in the Emergency with a wound to his mouth.

'Umm ... A piece of wood has cut through his lip, and my consultant said to call you to come and see it now.' Her voice quivered. A cut on the lip didn't sound too urgent so I told her I'd come and have a look once I'd finished my next case. A minute or so later, I got another call, this time from the ED consultant.

'I don't care about your fucking hand surgeries! You need to come here now! We have a man with a severe facial injury bleeding out of his face!' he yelled.

I kept my cool and said I'd be right over. When I got to the ED, the trauma bay was in chaos. An elderly gentleman had bandages all over his head. He was on blood thinners, so the bleeding had been hard to stop. A piece of wood had been flung towards his head from a mulcher and gone through his cheek straight into his mouth, ripping the gums off the bone.

As I started talking to him about the operation he would need to repair the damage, he slowly started to faint. I relayed to the Emergency staff that the priority after securing his airway would be to get an urgent CT scan of his brain. 'The facial injuries can wait. I can stitch his face back together once we know that he doesn't have a more serious head injury,' I said.

I power-walked down the labyrinth of corridors to the front desk of the operating theatre to inform the anaesthetist and nurse in charge about the trauma patient. Then I went back to my 'fucking' hand surgeries.

'Sorry everyone, I had to sort out a patient in ED,' I said as I walked back in and swung on my surgical loupes, which allowed me to see small structures at triple the magnification.

'Yes, he's coming here now,' said the scrub nurse setting up a trolley of instruments.

'What? But he needs a CT scan first,' I said.

'ED called a Code Crimson.'

'But why? The bleeding's stopped.'

'Apparently when they were trying to intubate him, they dislodged the clot and he started bleeding again,' called out the anaesthetic nurse, who was drawing up medications into syringes.

I wished that the ED consultant had rung me when the man started bleeding again rather than being trigger-happy with the Code Crimson. I was worried about this patient's brain; I did not want to operate on him without excluding a head injury first. I called Jack to talk to him about what was happening.

'That's a big case, Shinkansen,' said Jack, who had nick-named me after the Japanese bullet train for my efficiency. I wasn't a fan of cultural references, but most of the time I was too occupied with patients to care. Besides, Jack was Indonesian. It was confusing when comments like this came from a fellow Asian – did it make them less racist, or not racist at all?

'Yes, it's quite a nasty facial injury. But shouldn't we get a CT scan first?'

'I'm with the boss now,' he said. 'I'll talk to him.'

Jack rang me back after a few minutes. 'Dr Boyd says to proceed. I'm doing the elective operating list with him this arvo, but give us a yell if you get stuck.'

In the short time I had been at the hospital, my impression of Dr Boyd was that he didn't want to get involved in drama or politics, so I imagined he would've just said *sure, whatever, if ED wants the face fixed, then fix it*.

I could hear a commotion outside the theatre doors as the gentleman got wheeled in. I heard the urgency of the nurse's voice as she was handing him over, the beeping of his monitors, the wheels clunking down the corridor, and the sound of steam coming out of my ears. When I unwrapped his bandages I could see where the bleeding was coming from. A little spurt from the superior labial artery, near the upper lip. I asked for a 3-0 Vicryl tie. All those years of tying purple threads as a student always came back to me in these moments. I tied off the bleeding vessel.

'The bleeding has stopped. We can now take our time and proceed,' I said in my calmest voice. Inside, my own blood was doing circuits around my body at breakneck speed, but on the exterior I kept my cool. I deliberately washed my hands slowly under the warm water of the scrub sink to calm myself and prepare for the surgery. I kept thinking that this patient should really have gone to the CT scanners. Now he was here, it made sense for me to fix his face, but I was also mindful that I still didn't know what was happening inside his skull.

The facial injury was quite severe: I had to re-suspend his gums as if they were curtains. With nothing to sew them to, I passed the needle between his teeth and sutured the edge of his gums to the gum on the inside of his teeth. The procedure was finicky and time-consuming. It took me two hours to reconstruct his face.

As soon as I tied my last stitch I requested that the patient get sent to the CT scanners. I was pacing up and down the operating theatre waiting for his result. I opened the medical imaging page on the computer and kept pressing 'refresh' so that I could look at his scans as soon as they were uploaded.

As it turned out, he had a rather large subdural haemorrhage around his brain. Luckily for all of us his brain had atrophied with age, so his skull had enough space to accommodate the blood. That was a near-miss. My heart was overwhelmed with dread as I asked the switchboard operator to dial the neuro-surgical registrar. Would I get criticised for operating on the patient before he'd had a CT scan? Would I get yelled at even though I'd requested Emergency to get him the scan? Maybe I should have been more assertive. I wished I had more power. I wished I could have told the Emergency Department that I wouldn't accept this man until all the appropriate measures had been taken. But as an unaccredited registrar you couldn't do that. I was just glad the patient hadn't died.

Thankfully, the neurosurgical registrar seemed busy so he accepted my referral without asking any questions.

'I can't believe how calm you were throughout all that,' said the scrub nurse as I packed my bag to leave the operating theatre. I thanked her and walked towards the staff tea room feeling defeated. I couldn't have performed the surgery any better, but what's the use in performing surgery on a dead man? I hated that Emergency consultant for shouting and swearing at me, and for sending the patient to the operating theatre against my explicit instructions. And I hated myself for letting it bother me so much.

I sat down on a hard plastic couch in the tea room. The plastic had a crack in it, and bits of old, yellowed foam were crumbling out like stale lumps of sponge cake. I took my phone out of my pocket and scrolled through the news. My eyes stopped on a story that forced a quick, sharp gasp. A vascular surgeon, Dr Gabrielle McMullin, had made headlines over the weekend talking about sexism and harassment in surgery. The comment that had garnered the most attention was her saying, 'What I tell my trainees is that, if you are approached for sex, probably the safest thing to do in terms of your career is to comply with the request.' She referred to Ms Caroline Tan's sexual harassment case against her supervisor Dr Chris Xenos as a pyrrhic victory because Ms Tan had been blocked by her peers from securing a consultant role at any public hospital, limiting her work as a neurosurgeon to the private system. Dr McMullin commented that in terms of her career, Caroline, too, would have been better off giving Xenos a blow job and not complaining. That line made my gut twist. As outrageous as it sounded, I knew there was truth to it. The dirty, damning secrets of doctors have always been enshrouded by our professional code of silence, but now and then a crevice like this appeared.

An anaesthetist walked up to me in the tea room. 'We're ready for you in Theatre 3,' he said.

'Oh. I didn't think I had another case.'

'You were just talking to the patient.'

'I was? Which one?'

'The tonsil.'

Ah. He was talking about an ENT patient. He thought I was Jisoo.

Jack came into the tea room and sat down next to me. He must have finished his operating list with Dr Boyd.

'What you doing, Shinkansen?'

'I was just reading the story about Caroline Tan.'

'That lady surgeon in Melbourne?'

'Yes, the neurosurgeon who got sexually harassed.'

'Pretty dumb to complain about your boss,' Jack remarked. 'That's a sure-fire way to sabotage your career.'

I sat there unwilling to argue back. Was there any point in conversing with Jack about this topic? In that moment, he was the embodiment of Gabrielle McMullin's point, of the attitude that was hurting women in surgery.

Jack picked up a gossip magazine from the pile on the coffee table. A skinny blonde supermodel was on the cover. 'I'd tap that,' he said. 'That's totally my type. I like them anorexic-looking. I love when you can feel their bones.'

Only a few days later, another article in the paper stopped me in my tracks. A neurosurgeon in Melbourne had resigned over sexual harassment and bullying allegations. Kaufmann. That's all I could think of. Could it be? I sent Polly a text message straight away. My fingers couldn't have typed any faster. I needed to know. I wondered who the brave junior doctors were who'd banded together to file the complaint. A text message flew back from Polly. 'You bet. He's leaving the country.' *Wow*. Exiled. My heart was running a million miles. This was the first time I'd heard of a surgeon actually getting reprimanded for his behaviour.

When I got home that afternoon, I decided to go for a long run to shake off the icky feeling I had in my body. I felt really tense after the news that week. I knew that doing some form of exercise would reset and refocus me. I popped in some earphones and ran along the Parramatta River, watching the burned orange hues sink into the dark water.

That weekend, as usual, I went to my parents' home after a study session with Jisoo on Saturday morning. Mariko was still living at home and Eriko had just left for Japan. She was working in international disputes resolution at the Tokyo branch of an Australian law firm. After such an emotionally exhausting week I was extra grateful for Yoshiko's home cooking. As soon as I got there I flopped onto the couch like a rag doll and closed my eyes. Soon I was half-awake, half-asleep. Mariko was trying to converse with me but I was too tired to talk.

'Mummy,' I could hear her say. 'Yumiko's fallen asleep with her glasses on.'

'It's so she can see her dreams better, honey,' replied Yoshiko.

I couldn't help but smile at their cute exchange. I fell into a deep slumber and had a nightmare about the elderly patient with the facial trauma. I dreamed that when he woke up from surgery he'd had a massive stroke from bleeding into his brain. Recently, every dream I had was set in a hospital. When you work many hours, work follows you home, into your bed, and into your dreams.

25

Heartache

2015, Sydney

It was finally time for me to apply for the Program. I had put everything into my application, which was submitted in April. It was now May and I'd just received an email notification that my CV and references were enough to offer me an interview in June. I was one of eighteen candidates in New South Wales who had been shortlisted. Things suddenly felt more real. Jack emailed me some past interview questions to help me prepare, and even quizzed me between cases when we were in the operating theatre. He may have been a male chauvinist, but I was thankful that he was willing to help me out. For the weeks leading up to the interview, I practised every day, either with Jack or in front of the mirror at home. Jisoo helped me, too. The ENT questions were different from the Plastics ones, but we acted as mock interviewers for each other.

As a doctor in her fifth year of working, I felt it was well and truly time for me to take the next step and officially start specialty training. I was ready for the Program. I felt an intense pressure. Each day was like being at a concert with the bass booming so loudly that it reverberated through my skin to my organs.

As well as the hair and jewellery memo, I'd also heard that old-school surgeons expected women to wear skirt suits. Pant suits were a no-no. So on the day of the interview I wore a simple blouse underneath my black skirt suit and a pair of pearl earrings. And then I started to do my hair. After studying some YouTube videos and hair blogs, I'd perfected the chignon the day before, but it wasn't working that morning. For the last six years, I'd kept this mental note pinned to the corkboard in my head, but my hair was protesting. Wrestling with my lopsided chignon was a distraction from the main fight – that this was the most important interview of my life. Eventually I told myself to get a grip and I did my hair in a neat bun instead.

Having spent the previous four years away from Sydney, I walked into the interviews not knowing most of the other candidates. Nor did I recognise any of the consultant surgeons who were on the interview panel, which was a disadvantage. It put even more pressure on me to do well at this interview, because it would be based on first impressions. I hoped my personality and knowledge would come across favourably. I inhaled slowly and deeply, and drew my shoulders back.

The questions were all as expected. I answered them the best I could and left the interviews feeling cautiously optimistic.

The following weekend I was on call. I was handed over a patient who Rasheed had seen the day before, and was booked for a nail-bed injury. I undid the bandages on the patient's thumb to discover that he did not have a nail-bed injury at all. The tip of his thumb was amputated, hanging on by a thin strip of skin and totally unviable. In Medicine they say 'Don't trust anyone else's assessment of the patient.' I'd always reassessed all my patients, but this was the first time that a colleague had handed me over a patient with a grossly incorrect diagnosis.

I called Dr Boyd. I explained that the patient would need a flap to cover the tip of his amputation and I sent over a photograph of the wound then waited for him to call me back with a plan.

'Have you heard of a Segmüller flap?' he asked, referring to the surgeon who had pioneered the technique in 1976.

'Yes,' I replied confidently. 'It's a neurovascular island flap.'

'Good girl,' he said, and gave me one tip. 'Whatever you do, don't cut the nerves.'

Good girl. I hadn't been called that since primary school. Dr Boyd ended the call by saying, 'Call me if you need me,' which I had learned over the years to mean *don't call me unless you absolutely must.* A few minutes later, he sent a photo of his own thumb, on which he had drawn a triangle. 'Cut the flap out like this,' he captioned.

With the image Dr Boyd had sent etched on my mind, I walked into the operating theatre. I took off my glasses and replaced them with my magnifying loupes so that I could see the arteries and nerves in the patient's thumb. This, to me, represented the thing I loved the most about hand surgery – fine and detailed technique, resulting in a thumb that is reconstructed to look as close as possible to a normal, pre-injury thumb. With a scalpel, I cut the triangular flap on the patient's thumb, just adjacent to his wound, and then carefully dissected around his nerves and blood vessels with some scissors. I slid the flap into the defect at the top of his thumb and stitched it all together. At the end of the operation, I was proud of my handiwork. I took a picture of the flap and sent it to Dr Boyd, who replied with a 'thumbs up' emoji.

A few weeks later, I got a thumbs down. I did not get selected for the Program. I had spent all day checking my emails, and the bad news finally arrived at 3.30 pm. The candidates for the other surgical specialties who'd applied from the hospital had been notified first thing in the morning, so it was rather cruel to be at work all day surrounded by celebration while awaiting my fate. Every hour, a doctor or a nurse I was working with in the operating theatre or on the ward would enquire, 'So, any news?' 'How'd you go?' And each time I'd say 'Not yet,' and attempt to carry on with my day. It was excruciating. I knew they meant well but it wasn't helping. When I did receive the news, I was with Dr Boyd.

'You've got a good brain, good hands and a good heart,' he said. 'It didn't happen this year, but it will. Don't give up.'

I got a lump in my throat hearing those words from him. They were exactly what I needed. In a world like Surgery, where compliments were few and far between, his words stopped me from sinking into a deep dark hole. I was, of course, profoundly disappointed, but I knew I needed to get back up and keep going. I called Jisoo. She had narrowly missed out on a training position. She was ranked twelfth in the whole country, but the ENT training program was only accepting six registrars to commence training in 2016. She was so unlucky and I was devastated for her. In previous years she would have succeeded, but each year the number of positions was determined by how many final-year registrars passed their fellowship exams. For 2016 only those six positions were open in all of Australia.

There was little else Jisoo and I could do but resolve to focus on studying for the primary surgical exams. That reminded me to call Polly and Martha to see how they'd done with their resit examinations.

After work, I called Polly. Overall, her mark would have been enough to pass, but she had failed the Anatomy section by just half a point. You had to pass each section to pass overall, so Polly would have to retake the exam again. The next try would be her third and final. There was a rule that if you couldn't pass the primary exam within three attempts you'd be kicked off the Program. Imagine that. Working so hard to get on to the highly competitive training program only to get booted out at this stage. Martha, thankfully, had passed.

Having missed out on a position on the Plastics training program, I had to reapply for an unaccredited registrar position in August. That year, a centralised selection process for unaccredited plastic surgery registrar positions across Sydney had been introduced. You were offered an interview based on the strength of your CV. But once you were in the interview, the decision about jobs was solely based on what the panel thought of you, so there was an incredible amount of pressure on the day. The interview panel was huge. I sat in a board room across a large mahogany table, which was surrounded by a sea of suits – each representing one of the Sydney hospitals. Trish, a motherly, warm-natured woman from Medical Administration, offset the phalanx of fifteen men. I had twenty minutes to convince the room that I was worthy of a job for 2016. The questions were as expected. I wasn't sure whether I'd be allocated one of my top three choices but I was hopeful of a decent posting.

One of the rules was that we weren't allowed to be allocated a hospital we'd worked at before. Working at different hospitals was beneficial for our learning, as I already knew having moved back to Sydney from rural New South Wales. Unfortunately for me, the candidates who were ranked above me were allocated to all of the hospitals I hadn't been to before, leaving only my Western Sydney hospital. Since they couldn't reallocate me there, they gave my spot to someone ranked below me at the interviews and I was left without a position. How was it possible that someone ranked lower was offered a job, and I wasn't? I felt affronted by this decision, and then ashamed that I had failed to secure a job.

When Trish rang to deliver my outcome, we both felt powerless. She was merely the messenger. Sensing the despair in my voice, she offered to give me some feedback.

'I'm so sorry,' she said. 'Let me see if I can give you some information.'

'Thanks,' I replied. 'I just need to know where I went wrong. I thought my interview went well.'

'Right . . . Yumiko, Yumiko . . .' she said out loud as she flicked through her papers. 'Ah, here you are.' I held my breath. 'Well, it looks like most of the surgeons scored you between sixteen and eighteen out of twenty. A couple of them even gave you nineteen.'

'Okay . . .'

'But you got five from North Shore and Concord.'

'Five? Five!' My head was spinning. 'I don't understand how they could give me five when everyone else thought I was in the high teens. Did they write any comments?'

'No,' said Trish. 'Look, I don't know why you got that score. I really shouldn't be giving you this information, I'm sorry I can't say any more.'

'It's okay,' I said, although I was desperate for more information. I thanked her and hung up the phone. How was I ever going to get on to the Program if this was what happened at the unaccredited level? I was dumbfounded by the unfairness of it, and immediately stressed about potential unemployment.

I knew I couldn't possibly tell my parents. What would they think of me? They'd put me through medical school and now I was going to be an unemployed doctor. How shameful. I wallowed in self-pity as I thought about my decline. Two rejections within the space of a few months. They were huge blows to my confidence. This was the first time in my life that I'd felt like a failure. I was educated. I was qualified. I was passionate and hard-working. Yet I couldn't get a job in my chosen area.

Entering this liminal stage was disorientating. I was a doctor, sure, but without entry to the Program, I had no sense of security. And now I didn't even have an unaccredited registrar position. For the first time in my life I told myself: *you're fucked.*

Yoshiko rang me later that week. It was 9 pm and I was driving home from work.

'Yumiko, can you come and see Dad? He doesn't look right.' I could detect the worry in her voice even through the muffled Bluetooth system in my car. Yoshiko never asks for anything, so I knew she must be gravely concerned.

'I'll be there right away,' I said, as I shifted into the right lane and put my foot down on the accelerator.

When I got home, Dad was in my parents' room looking grey and a little sweaty, curled up on their futon in the foetal position.

'What's wrong, Dad?' I asked.

'Oh, I think it's just the cold-and-flu tablet I took this morning.'

'What's happening?' I probed.

'It just feels a bit heavy on my chest,' he said, still unmoving. I was starting to feel clammy myself, seeing my father like that.

'If it's been longer than fifteen minutes, we should go to the hospital,' I said.

'It's been an hour or so,' he said.

'Get up now. Put some clothes on, I'm driving you to the hospital.' I was now in commando mode. My heart started to race. This was a true emergency.

I found Yoshiko in the kitchen and told her we needed to go to the hospital immediately. 'I'll drop you off at the front of the Emergency Department and then go and park the car. Make sure you tell the triage nurse that he has chest pain,' I whispered as Dad was getting changed.

Yoshiko nodded and looked at me with worry in her eyes. I reassured her that it was going to be okay, although I wasn't sure of it myself.

With my lead foot we got to Royal North Shore Hospital in less than five minutes – much faster than if we had rung the ambulance, explained Dad's symptoms, and waited for it to come. Dad was cracking jokes all the way there, trying to defuse the tension in the car.

I pulled over at the entrance of the Emergency Department and grabbed Hajime's arm.

'Now, listen, Dad. You look at me. Stop. Making. Jokes. If you're carrying on like this, they're not going to take you seriously. You hear me? You clutch your chest, walk slowly like you're actually in pain. Can you do that?' I said, piercing his eyeballs with my glare.

'Okay,' he replied, sensing the gravity of the situation.

I watched Hajime stagger slowly towards the triage desk dramatically holding his hand against his chest, all the muscles on his face scrunching into a tense grimace. *Good job, Dad.* I drove off to find some parking and returned to find him already in a cubicle.

I recognised the intern who was looking after him – he was one of the medical students I'd taught Anatomy to many years before, which felt strange. One of my baby students had all grown up. *You can do it, Jim, look after Dad well . . .* I stepped out of the cubicle. The worst thing when you're trying to do your job is having a family member breathing down your neck, especially if that family member is a doctor. I didn't want to put any pressure on the staff, so I stepped back, and motioned Yoshiko to do the same.

Jim kept his professional face on, even if he did recognise me. He did a fine job introducing himself to Hajime and explained what he was going to do. Dad had his blood taken, and a trace of his heart. There was an anaesthetic registrar I recognised, too, who was standing by the doctors' station. I'd worked with him last year. We saluted each other with a short wave. He gave me a sympathetic look. Hajime had ST elevation on his ECG, which translates to a massive heart attack. A senior registrar came to deliver the news to him.

'What?' Hajime was in total disbelief. My heart broke for him. 'Oh, a heart attack? Really? I see . . .'

'Yes, it looks like a serious one, so we are going to move you to another bay where we can monitor you more closely. The cardiologist is on the way in.'

Yoshiko and I accompanied Dad as we moved over to the resuscitation bay. He was sent to the Catheter Lab shortly afterwards, where the offending blockage in his main coronary artery was cleared via a catheter threaded up to the heart from the groin.

Dad was lucky to be alive. Although he was a stoic man, it was clear to me that stress had caused his heart attack. He didn't have any other risk factors for heart disease. He didn't smoke, he wasn't obese, and his blood pressure and cholesterol had been normal. After losing his friend to overwork just a few years prior, Dad had nearly become a casualty of *karoshi* himself.

Hajime needed bypass surgery a week after his heart attack. After the surgery Yoshiko and I visited him in the ICU. I'd seen plenty of people in the ICU with breathing tubes, but this was my father. I tried to hold back the tears as I saw him propped upright in the patient bed, his eyes closed, his skin pale, and a plastic tube going down his throat. He looked like he was dead. I composed myself and sat beside him, holding his cold, limp hand. I knew he was too sedated to interact, but I also knew that people who were intubated could still sense things.

Yoshiko was strong throughout the next week, not once showing any distress. She took the train to and from the hospital every day and I think the routine kept her going.

A few nights after he'd first been admitted, Hajime went into rapid atrial fibrillation, which means the heart starts beating erratically at a really fast rate. Kind of like doing burpees at a boot camp, except you can't stop. Apparently it's terrifying and feels like you're going to die. It's fairly common after any sort of open-heart surgery – the heart's gone through a lot, so sometimes the stress of it all makes it go into a funny rhythm. I remember treating many of these on the ward. I would casually prescribe medications to slow down the rate, make sure the patient had good levels of magnesium and potassium, and then carry on with my shift like it was no bother. It felt different when it was actually my father. The night shift nurse who had looked after him overnight when it had first happened told me that Hajime wanted to write a farewell note. Even though she had reassured him that his heart was going to settle, Hajime had convinced himself that he was going to die, and had asked her for a pen and paper. She couldn't find a piece of paper, so he wrote on a paper towel:

Dear Yoshiko, Yumiko, Eriko and Mariko,
I love you very much. I am proud of you and all of your achievements. I leave all of my possessions to my wife, Yoshiko.
Hajime Kadota

Oh Dad . . . This was the first time he'd ever shown this kind of emotion. It was certainly the first time he'd told any of us he loved us. I could barely contain myself as I read it the next morning. I put the note into my handbag. By then Hajime was back to his normal spirits, telling us about how terrible the rapid AF felt. He was animated and gesticulating as he was describing it to us, and laughed it all off.

Over the course of the next few weeks Hajime had several bouts of AF. It was still frightening every time, but now that he knew he wasn't going to die from it, he learned to ride the wave.

After one of my visits to the Intensive Care, I received a phone call from a surgeon who'd been on the interview panel. He wanted to offer me a job as a Plastics registrar in the private system. I wasn't sure how I felt about that. Formal training takes place at public teaching hospitals, and there's a bit of a stigma working in a private hospital like the one he was talking about, where most of the work was cosmetic. I'm talking boob jobs, tummy tucks, and mummy makeovers – not exactly the altruistic reason I signed up for Medicine. Nevertheless, a job's a job. I would be working with two consultant Plastic Surgeons, Dr Grimshaw and Dr Whiteley. A couple of days a week they consulted at their private practice, and they spent the other days performing surgeries at a few different private hospitals. Although I was reluctant to take the role, I had no other options but unemployment. So I accepted, at least relieved that I didn't have to let my parents down.

In October, Jisoo and I sat the surgical primary exams. We were ready. It wasn't always easy to stick to the study schedule as we had our on-call responsibilities for work, but we managed to get a lot done throughout the year. When we couldn't physically catch up, we emailed each other our notes. It was a real team effort that we got through the enormous amount of content for the exam.

A few weeks later we received our results: we'd both passed. It was a mildly happy moment, more like relief that we wouldn't have to study anymore. I thought about my friends who had failed – it was a difficult exam. I knew I should have been prouder. The truth was, the exam didn't mean anything unless I got on to the Program.

At the end of the year, I was lucky enough to get Christmas Day off to spend time with my family. Rasheed and Asif were Muslim so they'd offered to work. It would be my last Christmas with Mariko in Sydney, as she had just accepted a job in Tokyo and would be moving back in the New Year to live with Grandma, who was now in her late eighties and needing more help around the house. Unlike Eriko, Mariko had decided not to become a lawyer, and instead to use her Commerce degree to work in corporate development services. I was proud of her for choosing her own path.

Mariko and I went for a run around our neighbourhood before settling in front of the telly. We put on the news on the Japanese channel, NHK. The usual visuals of the illuminated streets around Tokyo dominated the footage. However, there was one heartbreaking story that caught my attention. A twenty-four-year-old lady had committed suicide after working one hundred hours of overtime that month. Just a week before jumping off a building, she wrote on her Twitter account,

'When you're working twenty hours a day, you don't know what you're living for anymore. It's so pathetic. It's laughable.'

The sad thing was, I was used to this sort of news now. Japanese people work too hard. I told myself I'd never work in Tokyo. It sounded way too toxic.

26

et al.

At the start of 2016, I met Dr Grimshaw, the principal surgeon I'd be working with for the year, and Bev, his practice manager. Bev was slender, thanks to a diet of detox juices, and her face was expressionless from a generous dosage of *Botulinum* toxin. Her over-inflated lips blew me air kisses as she sashayed out of the room after our quick introduction. Dr Grimshaw sat me down to explain how the year would work. One day a week I would be in the private rooms assisting the nurse to review the post-operative patient's wounds and to take out any stitches. On the other four days I would be assisting in operations. The perks of the job would also include paid conferences and training courses, including a course to qualify me in injecting Botox and filler.

The world of injectables was foreign to me. Even though women can do whatever they want to their bodies, I was a little uneasy about this work. There was perhaps a bit of internalised misogyny at play: having never needed or wanted cosmetic work myself, I projected my belief in ageing naturally. More importantly, I knew that being a cosmetic injector wasn't going to be particularly helpful for my Program application, even though I liked the idea of learning some new skills.

Months went by and it was clear that the perks weren't going to happen – they simply never transpired and if I asked about a conference or training course, I was fobbed off. Dr Grimshaw was a nightmare to work with. 'Chop, chop, chop, chop, chop, chop, chop, chop, chop!' he would scream every time a suture needed to be cut, as though shouting at me would make me any quicker. He had a high turnover of nurses because no one wanted to work with him. Dr Grimshaw had no regard for the theatre nurses.

Initially, working in the private system meant I had a bit more time to exercise, and because of my frustration with work, I decided that I would try to offset it by training for a half-marathon.

One day a week, I assisted the other surgeon working at Dr Grimshaw's practice, Dr Whiteley. Dr Whiteley was relatively young and seemed to be interested in supporting other young female surgeons. She was softly spoken, polite, and never uttered a bad word about anybody. She had perfectly straightened hair and dressed meticulously in designer dresses. She looked out for me, as well as for Yoni, another female unaccredited registrar who also assisted her from time to time. Yoni was a striking woman with blonde curls and a strong, aquiline nose. She had piercing blue eyes, and her eyelashes were coated with black mascara. She split her time between a public and private hospital. Her contract and main obligation were with a public hospital, but the surgeons who worked there took her over to the private hospital whenever they needed assistance. Even though Dr Whiteley didn't have a public appointment, she had enough connections to be able to 'borrow' Yoni. Time is money. If plastic surgeons are able to finish their operations quicker with the help of an assistant, it means that they can do more operations in a day and earn more money. Taking registrars from their public hospital responsibilities to help surgeons with their private operations was frowned upon because registrars were paid by the public health system. It was a reverse Robin Hood scenario – or, more simply, stealing – but it was ubiquitous.

Soon after I met Yoni, we talked about the Program. I was ready to enter the fray for the second time. I'd done all four of the surgical courses offered through the Royal Australasian College of Surgeons (RACS), I had the right experience on my CV and I was now studying every night when I got home from the hospital, scrutinising past interview questions I had got hold of from Jack, and practising my responses. Both Dr Grimshaw and Dr Whiteley had long operating lists, which meant that soon I was working a lot of overtime hours till late at night, but I made sure that I still dedicated at least an hour a night to my interview preparation.

Yoni was also applying for the Program, and admitted to being terrible at interviews, so I offered to practise with her. She tended to mumble and came across as unsure of herself. I gave her all of the past questions I had, and we practised every week. I didn't know whether Yoni had good technical skills or not, but I strongly believed that there was enough space for both of us to succeed. Women should lift each other up, especially in a male-dominated field like Surgery where we're outnumbered and disadvantaged. Yoni and I became good friends, often meeting up for coffees and lunches to practise answering the questions. The interviews would be held in June and when we started our study together it was only April, so we had a good couple of months to prepare.

I enjoyed working with Dr Whiteley. I thought that in her maybe I would finally find a female mentor in Surgery. She'd had her challenges but she was now a successful plastic surgeon working in private practice. She had done a cancer-related PhD and aspired to specialise in it, but she was overlooked at the end of her training: instead a male surgeon was appointed to the position she'd applied for, despite her credentials and extensive research in the area. It seemed that even after qualifying as a specialist, getting a public hospital appointment was difficult. She didn't seem too bitter about it. She loved private practice and she had two kids to look after. Not having to be on call for the public hospital allowed her to spend a bit more time with her family, although her hours were still long.

One Friday in April we started operating at 8 am and the last procedure finished well after midnight. I was flying early the next morning to Melbourne for the Geelong half-marathon. I was looking forward to the event. Polly, my neurosurgery registrar from a few years ago, was coming to support me, as was May, who I hadn't seen since I'd been in Sydney.

I was exhausted when I arrived in Melbourne. I could barely stay awake as I took the Sky Bus into Spencer Street station in the city. There, I took the train to Geelong. Our accommodation was not ready for check-in yet so I couldn't rest. I dragged myself around Geelong, and decided to wait at the library, where I had a sneaky little nap. Polly and May arrived later that evening and we all went out for dinner. It was great to introduce them to each other, and have a good time, the three of us. Working in the private practice was not very social because I only really saw Dr Grimshaw and Dr Whiteley.

The next morning I had to get up early for the race. I was still very tired from the working week, and a little dehydrated. I regretted having any wine the night before, albeit just a glass. Nevertheless, I fronted up to the start line. I'd never run feeling so exhausted and I resented that long Friday I'd worked. My body was letting me down and I knew I was running much more slowly than usual. I kept drinking water around the course. Rookie error. It made me vomit at the 19-kilometre mark. After that short disruption I managed to run the final couple of kilometres but I wasn't happy with my time at all.

I was feeling disgruntled about everything. Despite working in the private system, which didn't have any on-call responsibilities, I was still working long hours. I wasn't receiving the right experience for my future, and I wasn't really enjoying the work. I missed the feeling I got when I performed hand surgery, whether it was perfectly realigning a broken bone, or reconstructing the tip of an injured finger.

On the Monday back at work Dr Grimshaw spoke to me about a reference chapter he'd been meaning to write. When he'd spoken at a conference the previous year, he had been invited to contribute to an upcoming surgery publication. My eyes lit up. The opportunity to get published in a book was a lot harder to come by than a journal article. In fact, when I thought about my colleagues, the only person I recalled authoring something similar was a girl whose father was a well-respected Emergency physician. I remember seeing their names together, a reminder that having family contacts conferred such an advantage at times.

'Let me send you the letter from the publisher,' said Dr Grimshaw, as he opened up his inbox. 'What's your email address again?'

Despite his surgical dexterity, Dr Grimshaw couldn't type quickly. As I watched him tap out my address with just his two index fingers, one letter at a time, I realised why he had been putting off writing the chapter. At his speed, it would take him years.

Later that morning, one of Dr Grimshaw's secretaries approached me. It turned out that while I was on a measly salary and not getting paid any overtime, Dr Grimshaw was charging patients an assistant fee by the hour for my work. I spoke to Dr Whiteley about this discovery and she was horrified. She thought that Dr Grimshaw would have at least given me some time off in lieu for all the extra hours. She didn't have much power in the matter as she was sub-contracting, but she started to pay me by the hour for my time.

Dr Whiteley knew what was involved in getting on to the Program so I also asked her whether she'd start doing some mock interviews with me at work to prepare for the selection interviews. Last year, around twenty of us had been short-listed for the interview, but I was one of just nine this year in New South Wales. Included in the nine were Trevor and Yoni.

After I'd been shortlisted, I found out that Dr Whiteley was giving Yoni some extra practice sessions on weekends. On one occasion she invited Yoni to her home and held a mock interview for her with another senior plastic surgeon whom Yoni worked with in the public hospital. When Yoni told me about it I was really upset. This was everything I'd worked for. Six years of medical school. Six years of working as a doctor. I didn't understand why Dr Whiteley was helping Yoni but not me, her private assistant and, I thought, her mentee.

'You don't need any help,' Dr Whiteley explained.

'I do! I need all the help I can get,' I said.

'I'm more worried about Yoni. I know you'll be all right.'

I wasn't sure I was buying it. Something didn't feel right to me. Why did she favour Yoni? I helped Dr Whiteley every single week with her operations, often working late into the night. We got along like sisters. Was I missing something here? I wondered whether it was to do with the other plastic surgeons whom Yoni was working with. From what she had described in our chats over the last few weeks, her bosses all seemed very supportive of her. Perhaps they were pushing for her place on the Program, and Dr Whiteley was being recruited to this plan. It made me disheartened that there wasn't a similar push for me.

Nevertheless, I stuck my head down and continued interview practice on my own, and worked on the reference chapter. When I was done with the writing, I added some diagrams and clinical photographs I had taken with Dr Grimshaw's professional camera. And yet, when it came to submitting to the publishers, Dr Grimshaw insisted on being the first author, even though I had done the writing and put together the illustrative material. It was customary for the person who wrote the manuscript to be the first author, and that senior author was the final author. The ethics of authorship were well known to all doctors, so this was an awkward situation to be in. I felt like I couldn't say anything, however, because without Dr Grimshaw I wouldn't even have had this opportunity, and I needed it for my CV. So I did as he requested. For years to come, the reference chapter will be cited as Grimshaw *et al.* I am a nobody. I am invisible. I am '*et al*'.

27

Search Engine Optimisation

2016, Sydney

It was the end of June. The big interview day. I was wearing a silk white blouse, the same black skirt suit as the year before; my hair was in a chignon; and I had the pearl earrings on. I knew I looked the part. Now it was time for me to show the interviewers that I was an intelligent, confident, worthy candidate for the Program.

We were grouped in threes. I was in the same group as the daughter of one of the eminent surgeons in Sydney and I felt a bit defeated before the interview had even started: one of our interviewers was well known to be her father's best friend. They had worked together for decades at the same hospital and always sat next to each other at meetings and conferences. I wondered if I'd be differentially marked down and she marked up to make sure that she got on to the training scheme.

In a neighbouring interview room was another prominent plastic surgeon. He asked me about the research I'd done. The first answer that sprang to mind related to the material I had written for Dr Grimshaw.

'Doesn't count! It won't be peer-reviewed,' he interjected.

'Okay, well, I presented research at a conference in Barcelona,' I said.

'Has it been published in a journal?' he asked.

'No,' I replied, and looked down at my lap.

'Have you submitted it to any journals?'

'Yes, I have, but it hasn't been accepted by any yet,' I explained.

'If your research is so interesting, why do you think it hasn't been published?' he asked, staring at me, unblinking.

'I don't know,' I replied, feeling defeated.

To my relief, a kinder surgeon sitting next to him took over the questions. The rest of that round was a bit of a blur. I didn't feel optimistic about the result. At the end of the interview, I realised that all of the questions we'd been asked were included in the list Yoni and I had practised from; the list that I'd sent her. I wondered whether it was a mistake to have helped her.

We would have to wait an agonising month for the outcome of the selection process to be announced. In the meantime, Dr Grimshaw was off on a sojourn to Italy. Since there wouldn't be any of his surgeries to assist, Bev decided to allocate me some office work while he was away. She filled my inbox with a list of administrative and IT tasks to complete:

1. SEO for the practice website
2. Spell and grammar check every page on the website

3. Two or three blog posts for the website
4. Disaster Management Plan for when the IT system goes down

What the hell was SEO? I scrolled through all of the other emails Bev had sent me, each a few minutes apart. There were ten emails about Search Engine Optimisation. Ah. And a disaster management plan? That seemed like a highly specialised computer-y thing to do. I was mortified that this was what I was having to do while I waited for arguably one of the most important results of my career.

And then the following day, while I was working on the practice's website, I noticed a photograph in one of the files. The harsh interviewer. I felt my stomach churn as I relived my interview with him. I couldn't believe he was a former practice partner of Dr Grimshaw. I asked the secretaries about him and they told me that he'd had some sort of falling out with Dr Grimshaw, and they were no longer on speaking terms. It was now clear that mentioning my writing with Dr Grimshaw was not going to have worked in my favour. *Oh well, there's nothing I can do now*, I told myself.

To break up the monotony of working on a computer every day, I ran. My body clock still woke me up at 5.15 each morning, so I would catch the train to Circular Quay and run in the Botanic Gardens, being chased by the laser beam sunrise. It was a beautiful way to start the day, and made the office work a bit more tolerable.

I thought I'd better make the best of this ridiculous situation I'd been left in, so, having always enjoyed writing, I decided to get on with a couple of blog posts for the practice website. Not that I'd ever have admitted it to Bev, but I did find writing the posts kind of fun. I fiddled with a few tags to improve their SEO.

In July I was informed that I hadn't got a place on the Program. Unsuccessful. Try again next year. It was the same text as the year before, just copied and pasted with a 2016 time-stamp. I stared at my computer screen and absorbed the bad news. I was gutted. My colleagues were talking about who got on and who didn't. Yoni and Trevor had made it through. I never heard from Yoni again. She didn't need me anymore. I let my referees know about my result. Some were outraged and suggested I contact RACS for further feedback. I was desperate for some answers so I did end up emailing the college, but an automated response was sent back to me that they were unable to release any referee marks or my interview score. They must have been inundated with similar emails from other candidates like me who were devastated and wanted closure. As a private entity, the Freedom of Information Act did not apply to RACS. With no clues as to why I had been rejected, I was left in a state of despair, like I'd been ghosted. I had worked hard over the preceding six years to obtain good references, gain clinical experience and maximise my points on the CV. I presented myself well and thought that I had answered the questions well at the interview. What more did I have to do?

I rang Jisoo, hoping that she had made it on to ENT, but to my shock and disappointment she too had been rejected. She was taking it even harder than I was. She'd been so close yet again – like the previous year, she'd missed out by just a few places.

'I've decided to stop trying,' she said. Her voice sounded hollow.

'You can't, Jisoo! Don't give up. I know you're going to get on next year,' I said, trying my best to cheer her up. But she had made up her mind. She was going to apply for General Practice. Her boyfriend, Jun, wanted to be a surgeon too. He'd got on to the Urology training program. They decided that it would be too hard on their relationship for both of them to train in Surgery, so Jun would continue and Jisoo would become a GP. I could understand their decision. Surgical registrars work such long hours that if both of you did Surgery, you'd never see each other. I couldn't think of too many surgeons who were coupled up with another surgeon. I wondered what would have happened if Jisoo had got on to the Program and Jun hadn't, though. Would Jun have made the same sacrifice?

To cope with my disappointment, I continued to run. A lot. Every Sunday I'd go for a long run around the Botanic Gardens. I needed a new short-term goal to make myself feel better, that I wasn't a complete failure. I felt like a nobody. *Until I'm on the Program, I'm not officially anything.* I decided that I would run my first marathon in September. Then at least I could call myself a marathoner, I thought. I had five weeks, and I was determined. Forty-two kilometres. I gave myself no choice but to do it. *Just do it, Yumiko. You need to do it for you.*

One afternoon, I was walking from Darlinghurst to Town Hall station, past the Starbucks on the corner of Elizabeth and Park streets. Out of habit, I looked inside, and had to do a double-take. It was the ex-MedSoc president, Bill, serving coffees. Bill was a fifth-year medical student when I was the first-year rep. I looked up to him, like I did all senior medical students. What was he doing as a barista? I stared wide-eyed for a moment before I kept going. It had been nearly a decade since I'd seen Bill at medical school. I wondered what had happened to him. While he may have ascended the MedSoc leadership ladder to presidency, I guess he didn't continue his medical career. I was shaken.

I knew I needed to reset and think about how I would approach my Program application for next year. I thought hard about what I needed to do to better myself as a candidate. Fortuitously, I was contacted by Dr Boyd because he needed me back in Western Sydney. The team was feeling overwhelmed with the workload and could use another registrar. I knew that continuing to work for Dr Grimshaw was not doing me any favours. Assisting cosmetic surgery procedures was not helpful for this stage of my learning and training. I needed to re-immerse myself into the public health system and look after patients with trauma and disease. I needed to find my sense of purpose again. My *ikigai*.

I was re-hired in Western Sydney for some part-time work and I left Dr Grimshaw's practice. He was not happy at all. I did keep in touch with Dr Whiteley and as I would only be working part-time in Western Sydney, I continued to assist her surgeries.

It seemed important to remain committed to educational activities, and I did enjoy discussing the latest surgical literature, so later that week I decided to attend the Plastic Surgery Journal

Club in the CBD for the first time. When I got there, I saw a glowing Trevor. I wanted to hide out of embarrassment but I tried my best to put on a genuine smile and congratulate him.

'Look, don't feel bad for not getting picked,' he said smugly. 'The panel already know who they want to choose before the interviews.'

I thought back to the surgeon's daughter in my group. I really didn't want to give credence to his statement, but *was* there truth in it?

'Besides,' he continued, 'look at who gets on. You need to be blonde.'

He laughed. Trevor was half joking but when I looked around the room, I was the only Asian female there. All the other women were indeed blonde. Trevor smiled and sat down. The uppity air around him was unbearable. I chose a seat on the other side of the room.

28

It's a marathon, not a sprint

2016, Sydney

Spring was approaching in Sydney. I loved this time of year. Having grown up in Singapore, I never got used to the cold, even though winters in Sydney are mild and probably warmer than London summers. Spring made me feel hopeful. The jacarandas were budding. There's nothing quite like jacaranda blossoms – I always looked forward to the bursts of amethyst adorning the tree-lined streets of suburbia.

On the Sunday of the Sydney marathon, I felt inspired. I was running to raise money for a brain tumour charity that was close to my heart, and had already raised $4000. I decided to run my first marathon as a fairy. I woke up early to put face paint on, and sprayed my hair silver. My pre-race preparation felt almost surgical: I picked up little silver stars with my DeBakey forceps, applied a small amount of Dermabond skin glue and placed the stars onto my skin, forming a constellation on my cheeks. Then I stuck some metallic purple lashes onto my lids. I wore my hand-sewn tutu and carried a purple wand with a star on the end. After pinning some little angel wings to the back of my top, I was ready. The complex hair and make-up regimen calmed me by distracting me from the forty-two kilometres I was about to run.

'Big night last night?' a voice called out to me in the mosh pit of runners disembarking at Milsons Point train station. I laughed as the jovial crowd moved in one fluid mass out through the ticket barriers. I was a little self-conscious of my fairy costume among the sea of serious Lycra – wearing a tutu to a marathon made me feel like I was really putting the 'moron' in oxymoron. Why couldn't I be normal and just have worn compression gear? I tried to soak in the electric atmosphere underneath the Sydney Harbour Bridge.

I decided to run with a pacing group, which helped me maintain a steady tempo. The adrenaline must have helped because I didn't feel much pain for most of the race. Towards the end, as we approached Sydney Harbour, the salty air made my skin chafe. It irritated me, but I kept going. I felt strong. My physical preparation wasn't perfect, but I knew I had the mental strength to finish.

The overwhelming high I felt as I crossed the finish line was incomparable. Running a marathon was the greatest experience of my life. When I crossed that line, I was as elated as I've ever felt. And I completely forgot about feeling a loser for not getting selected on to the Program. In that moment I became a marathoner and no one could take that away from me.

The comedown from my marathon high, however, was abrupt. Hajime had had a biopsy. I didn't even know he had a lump in the first place, but it turned out that he'd barely recovered from his heart attack when he felt a lump in his groin. As usual, my parents did not want to worry my sisters and me, so the biopsy results were the first I heard of his discovery. I was worried for him – he just couldn't get a break – but I tried to keep positive. Lumps don't necessarily mean cancer. It could be an infection. Yoshiko was of course by his side when he went to the GP to find out.

The pathology report revealed that his lump was a lymphoma, and he was referred to a cancer clinic at the Royal North Shore Hospital. Luckily, it was a slow-growing type of tumour. However, this meant that he wasn't triaged as a priority so it would be several months before we could get in to see an oncologist. Poor Yoshiko was very anxious about the wait. I tried to reassure her to have faith in the triage system, and that it was a good thing Hajime didn't need an urgent appointment. It meant it wasn't as serious as other cancers.

The year was throwing up a lot of stuff I'd hoped not to have to face. I tried every day to stop my failure to get on to the Program from eating away at my confidence or getting me down too much. I was working as hard as I could at the hospital, partly to lose myself in the operations, which also helped me to forget my dad's plight, and partly to show myself and the staff there what I was capable of. I was getting faster and faster at fixing hand fractures, and gaining a good reputation among the theatre staff. I even ended up operating on one of the nurses – on a broken finger she'd sustained during a game of Oztag – and on the son of one of the other nurses, who had broken his hand in a rugby tackle. To me, this was the best compliment I could receive as a registrar – that my colleagues trusted me enough to let me operate on them, or their loved ones.

At the end of jacaranda season I was invited to a Christmas party on the harbour held by Dr Boyd. It was a perfect Sydney summer's day. The sun created crystals on the water, and the sand shone like glitter. I wore a light blue dress and my hair was down. I brought my DSLR to the party so that I could be the unofficial photographer. There were a few plastic surgeons, nurses, and staff from my Western Sydney hospital, as well as some doctors who worked in private practice. I sat on a bench to play with the settings on my camera to adjust for the sunlight streaming in from the opposite direction.

'Maxence de Beaumarchais,' a man said. I looked up to find him holding out his hand. I recognised his face. He was a well-known Sydney plastic surgeon.

'Oh, hello, I'm Yumiko,' I replied with a firm handshake to make sure I came across confidently.

The man stood there in fine Italian cotton shorts, a polo shirt and boat shoes. His steely blue eyes squinted into the sun and he brushed his fingers through his silver hair. On his arm was a stunning woman, with luscious locks cascading past her shoulders. She looked like a beauty queen in a white broderie anglaise dress, oversized sunglasses and some wedge espadrilles on her dainty feet. She left to join the other WAGs of plastic surgeons at the bar for a glass of champagne.

'I hear your suturing's neat and fast,' he said.

'Oh, thank you, Dr de Beaumarchais. I'm sure I'm just average,' I replied.

'Call me Max. I'll get my secretary to get in touch if I ever need an assistant.' He flashed his pearly whites and disappeared into the crowd.

Since I was only working part-time in Western Sydney, I was keen to pick up some work assisting surgeries. I wasn't expecting the Christmas party to be a networking opportunity, but I was glad to have met a new surgeon I could potentially work with.

Sure enough, I did hear from Maxence's secretary the following week and she offered me some work. I spent the following few months assisting Maxence when I was available. He was a specialist breast surgeon, and one of the best in Sydney by reputation.

Maxence was the most meticulous surgeon I'd met. The first operation in which I assisted him felt like an audition. 'Yumes can close the wound,' he said. 'Take your time; make it perfect.'

His scrub nurse, Daisy, handed me a pair of fine-toothed Adson forceps and a 4-0 Monocryl suture. The instruments had gold handles on them. Only the best equipment for the best surgeons in town. I could see two sets of eyes watching my every stitch. I made sure my hands were stable, and that my suturing was precise.

After closing the wound, Daisy smiled at me. 'Very neat,' she said.

Maxence inspected my work. 'Very good, Yumes. Looks almost like I did it.'

One day, a few months into my time helping Maxence, I was in the staff kitchen flipping through the paper when I nearly spilled my tea. A headline inside the paper read, 'Oncologist jail

261

term for drugging, assaulting colleague slashed'. My tea started sloshing in its cup. It was strange to see my hands shaking – they were usually very steady, but I couldn't control them. I couldn't concentrate on the words on the paper – they were about Dubia. He had gone to jail? He'd assaulted someone else? I'd clearly missed his original sentencing.

I did some frantic googling on my phone and found out that he'd been jailed the previous year. I wasn't interested in the news around that time – I was spending all my free time training for the marathon. Three years before that, he had drugged a registrar and she'd woken up to him sucking on her nipple. I could not believe what I was reading. Even though I knew firsthand the kind of man Dubia was, I had not thought him capable of something that awful – all-out assault. He'd drugged this woman for sex!

So many thoughts were whizzing through my head – a mixture of disgust at his behaviour, and guilt. Maybe I should have put in a formal complaint when I was his student a decade ago. I recalled the barriers. And about what had happened to Caroline Tan reporting her supervisor. She was a fully qualified surgeon when she did so and her career was ruined by her speaking up. As a medical student I was naïve and vulnerable. Was I supported or encouraged to speak up when I reported Dubia's behaviour towards me? I didn't feel I had been.

I wondered how many victims of his there might have been in the past ten years. Dubia had been protected by the system all those years, with none of us daring to call him out, and now even the law seemed to be protecting him! It was deplorable. The article reported that his sentence had been shortened because of his 'outstanding' work in the medical community prior to his psychological decline. How did that have anything to do with the fact that this man was a predator? And how was his depression relevant to what he'd done? I'm not a psychiatrist but having depression did not seem an excuse for his long pattern of behaviour. He'd even written the victim a letter blaming his actions on work stress.

I read the victim impact statement. She said, 'I have read the thick folder containing the psychiatrists' reports and character references and I am again reminded of the power imbalance.' As a prominent medical figure, Dubia would have had a lot of friends in high places. The victim knew that she was at risk of being labelled a 'troublemaker', and she said in her statement that she was told on several occasions she'd be the one to lose the trial. It was a heartbreaking read. She said, 'the constant intrusive thoughts and questions about why I was chosen to be the victim of such a despicable crime have robbed me of my confidence and self-worth . . . I still feel the same rage, shame, and desire to just disappear.'

My head was dizzy from the potent cocktail of shock, relief, anger and guilt shaken together in an emotional mixer. By the time I'd finished reading the article, I was shivering and my tea had gone cold. I walked back into the operating theatre readying myself for the next case, but inside I was still seething. The idea of what the registrar had suffered at that man's house that night, and what she must be going through now, haunted me for months.

29

Rainbows and unicorns

2017, Sydney

At the start of 2017, Hajime finally received an appointment with the oncologist for his lymphoma. This time I insisted that I go with him and Yoshiko to the hospital so I could help him understand all the medical jargon. I knew from my studies that when patients go to appointments – especially if they have a fraught diagnosis like cancer – they can often feel overwhelmed and forget half the information they're given.

The oncologist told Hajime that he had several options for treatment, but their utility would depend on whether the cancer had spread. If the cancer were just in the groin, it was treatable with radiotherapy. He was referred for a PET scan to see whether the lymphoma had metastasised. He had this scan a week later, which unfortunately showed that the cancer had spread above his diaphragm to lymph nodes under his arms. This meant that it was untreatable with radiotherapy. Instead, his oncologists would monitor him every few months with scans. He would be offered chemotherapy if the cancer troubled him with any symptoms, but it would not be curable. The doctors reiterated that this was a slow-growing lymphoma, so Hajime would still have several years to live. I looked at Hajime's face as he was listening to his doctor. He was visibly shaken.

Over the coming weeks, Hajime's temperament and behaviours changed. I noticed that he was being a bit more affectionate towards us. He was also becoming more health conscious; eating more vegetables and going for long walks. He had dropped his hours at work after his heart attack, and now he decided that he and Yoshiko would move back to Japan, where he planned on continuing some part-time work.

I respected Hajime's decision even though I didn't know much about the health-care system in Japan. I knew that Australia's cancer care was excellent and part of me wanted him to receive treatment here. I also wanted to be close by just in case his health was to deteriorate. However, Hajime had already made up his mind. I think there were multiple factors that my parents considered. Grandma Naoko was close to ninety so Yoshiko wanted to be closer to her, and my sisters were already in Japan. They knew I'd be fine alone in Australia. I'd always been the strong, independent one. They were right. I did feel fine. I was too focused on work to get sentimental about their move, anyhow. Hajime and Yoshiko left for Tokyo at the end of March, just in time for the cherry blossoms.

In August, I started work at the Children's Hospital. The Plastics team there looked after children with burns and hand injuries, as well as performing operations on babies born with cleft lip or cleft palate, and skull deformities.

There was something magical about working in a kids' environment. Every colour of the rainbow brightened up the hospital walls, there were toys, play therapists who would come to entertain the kids, and everyone just seemed to be cheerful. The consultants were lovely, as you'd expect of surgeons who want to work with kids. I particularly warmed to Uncle Phil, as I'd soon grow to call him. Uncle Phil loved story time. Whenever the other two registrars and I would scrub into a case with him, he always had a funny or interesting anecdote to tell us. He said we were the reason he loved working at the public hospitals, because he loved to mentor. I liked his no-nonsense approach to things. What you see is what you get with Uncle Phil. After some disappointing experiences over the last few years, Uncle Phil restored my faith in the surgical profession, and made me feel as though I could really thrive in this nurturing environment.

I was working with an accredited registrar, Bernadette, and Caleb, who was unaccredited. Caleb was a short and skinny clone of Channing Tatum – the number of nurses swooning over him was a testament to that. Even after the disappointments of last year, to my relief I didn't feel inferior to Bernadette. It helped that Uncle Phil treated the three of us the same. We were all deserving of teaching and mentoring, regardless of how ahead (or behind) we were in training. I really admired his surgical approach because he didn't over-complicate things. Every decision he made was justified, and he was efficient. I liked that about his approach.

I was used to only the accredited registrar being tested across the operating table, but one day I found Uncle Phil testing me. And I was answering the questions correctly, which buoyed my confidence. I wasn't the only one to notice. At the evening handover, the resident teased me about being Uncle Phil's favourite, and Bernadette mumbled something under her breath about how she didn't get asked any questions by him that day.

I knew that sometimes Bernadette would go to the library to cry. She had children whom she never saw because she was always at the hospital working or studying. She watched videos of her kids that her nanny sent each day. Sometimes, if it wasn't too busy on the wards or in the operating theatres, I'd sit and watch the videos with her. I still couldn't imagine what it would be like to work in Surgery while being a mother. It was hard enough doing it as a single woman.

Bernadette was much loved by the patients and their parents. She would spend hours talking to parents, explaining things, reassuring them, giving them support and having a friendly chit-chat as though time were not an issue. In many ways she was the opposite to me. I just wanted to get things done as quickly as possible, while she liked to take her time. There was probably a happy medium between the two. Through observing Bernadette, I think I became better at talking with parents. I worried that in a children's hospital I would be overwhelmed by the stress of parents, their demands, expectations and the pressure that came with that. Actually, it ended up being something I enjoyed a lot about working with kids. I learned to be a doctor who parents – and, in subsequent rotations, relatives – could trust, and that's something I worked hard to cultivate during my time there.

On my first day on call at the hospital, I saw a twelve-month-old baby who had placed her pinky into a blender when her mother had taken her eye off her for a few seconds. The mother was absolutely devastated because the pinky was hanging on by just a piece of skin. The finger was tiny. I'd put back together a fifteen-month-old's pointer finger a few years before, but this was even smaller. I knew I had to call in the consultant, Dr Field. I hadn't worked with him before so I was nervous about calling him, and apologetic about bothering him, but to my surprise he was supportive and said he'd come in – 'no problems'.

I started the case when Dr Field was nearly at the hospital. The broken finger was not an issue for me, having fixed many broken bones with K-wires in the past few years. The challenging part would be the microscope work. Dr Field walked in just in time for the start of the microsurgical repairs. The nerve was so minuscule that it made the suture look like fisherman's rope. With Dr Field looking at my handiwork under ten times the magnification, there was a lot of pressure. As I tied the last knot together on the nerve, he gave me the proverbial pat on the back. 'You're really good at micro,' he said. It was a strange experience. Compliments were unusual in surgery, and supervision even more so. It was crazy that I thought like that. By now I had got so used to operating independently that having senior support felt like a luxury – even for something as complex as a partial amputation of a baby's finger.

From the start of term, I was keen to work on my application for this year's Program. I needed more research publications on my CV, and was grateful when one of the other consultants, Dr Bruno, asked me to write an article with him. Dr

Bruno had an interest in breast cancer and had a paper to write about the various options for breast cancer reconstruction. It was a complex and interesting area because one has to keep in mind the fact that some women require radiotherapy as part of their overall treatment, which can affect the viability of tissues with which to reconstruct. I started reading widely on the topic straightaway to get a good grasp of the current evidence in the surgical literature.

I got into work one morning to hear that Bernadette, who had been on call the night before, had been informed about a twelve-year-old boy called Harry, from a small town outside of Sydney, who'd had a bullet ricochet into his face. His friend was playing with his father's gun inside a caravan and accidentally fired it, hitting Harry. Bernadette hadn't come in because the boy's condition was stable, so as I was on call that day it was my duty to follow him up. I was a little rattled – it's not every day that you see a child with a gunshot wound in Sydney. But it was reassuring that Uncle Phil was the consultant on call, so I knew he'd help me, whatever happened.

Harry was indeed stable but the bullet had travelled through his shoulder into his face, so the poor boy was lying on a bed with three holes in his body. The bullet had shattered his jawbone. All I had to do was text Uncle Phil when the operation was taking place and he was right there to help me with it. The complex thing about this case, however, was not so much the physical wounds as the psychological trauma. The little boy was starting to have flashbacks, and his parents were understandably worried.

Harry recovered from the surgery, and I knew the wounds would heal well, but I wanted to make sure we prevented him from developing post-traumatic stress disorder. That was my biggest worry for him. I contacted the Trauma Clinical Nurse Co-ordinator to discuss a referral to psychological services close to the patient's town. Unfortunately, we were not on the same page.

'He doesn't need psychology follow up,' she said.

'But he's having flashbacks. He's got early signs of PTSD,' I replied.

'He's been assessed and cleared by social work. He doesn't need any more involvement from us. All right?'

I found the conversation a hard one. I thought about this boy's future; of young girls and boys who had unresolved trauma and how that can increase the risk of chronic mental illness, juvenile delinquency, dropping out of school, and other problems later in life. I felt a responsibility not to let this happen to my patient, and at that moment I felt that the hospital system was letting him down. He'd had a bullet fired into his face! Even an adult would be traumatised from such an accident. I confided in Uncle Phil about how disappointed I was.

'You gotta let the kid go,' he said.

'But isn't it our responsibility to make sure he has adequate psychological follow-up?'

'You've done everything you can. If Trauma says no, you gotta accept it.'

I looked at the white wall of the operating theatre, wondering how I could possibly discharge this boy back to his rural town with no support.

'Destiny,' said Uncle Phil. 'What will happen will happen. You can't control everything.'

I started to tear up. He looked over and saw my eyes, and gave me a side hug.

'I didn't upset you, did I?' he asked.

'No, no, it's nothing you said. I'm just . . . I'm just worried for this patient, that's all. I'll go and talk to his parents and discuss their discharge plan,' I said, and excused myself.

I walked into the empty corridor outside of the operating theatre and let myself cry for a few minutes. I was devastated at having to discharge Harry. Over the next weeks, despite what the Trauma CNC had told me, I went about organising psychological support, much to the relief of Harry's parents. I gave them my work email and kept in touch, asking how he was going back at home, and if there were any symptoms that they were worried about. I spoke to his school principal about his reintegration, and I was touched that the principal put in so much time and thought into how the school could best support the little boy's transition back into class. Being situated in a rural town, the school had only periodic access to professional counsellors, but the principal contacted the Department of Education to see if they could have special provisions. I was relieved to hear that while the Department of Health had failed them, the Department of Education did not. I kept my patient's GP in the loop, and also suggested some trauma-sensitive counsellors who could help in the area.

That day, having talked to Uncle Phil, I walked down the rainbow-coloured corridors of the Children's Hospital, with my unicorn torch swinging with my ID badge, and realised that maybe it wasn't all rainbows and unicorns here. Maybe I had to be the unicorn sometimes.

As 2017 came to an end, so did my time at the Children's Hospital. Since my family was in Japan, I offered to work Christmas to give Bernadette and Caleb time with their families. Bernadette was in charge of the roster and put me on call for a week, with Caleb as my back-up if things got hectic.

It didn't take long for me to be inundated with phone calls. At one point I was getting calls every five minutes, and most nights I was getting rung until 1 or 2 am. By the end of the week I was exhausted. I rang Caleb to see if he could cover my calls for a few hours so I could finish some paperwork, go and see my patients and even maybe grab a micro sleep. He didn't pick up his phone, so I sent him a text message. I went to the ward to check up on a young boy with a severe infection in his thigh. He'd received a bright yellow truck from Santa. We played with his truck and then I changed his dressings.

'You look tired,' his mum said.

'Oh, do I?' I asked, knowing full well how I looked.

'Thank you for looking after my son,' she said.

'It's my pleasure,' I said. 'I'm glad Santa knew you were here.'

I checked my phone. Still nothing from Caleb. My eyelids felt rough against my eyeballs. I desperately wanted a nap. I rang Caleb again but the phone rang out.

The next afternoon he sent me a text. He'd left his phone at a mate's place. Frustrating. What was the point of having this system if the back-up person was uncontactable?

I had the Monday night off but was back on call on the Tuesday. By Wednesday I was so tired I went to the library and slept on one of the couches. It was my tenth day in a row of work. There was something a bit ballsy about surreptitiously grabbing a nap where people around me were tapping away on their laptops or studying, but there weren't many other places I could sleep at the hospital. Caleb came to wake me up at lunchtime; it was time for the clinic. To my great relief, Uncle Phil saw how tired I was and suggested I take Friday off. I was grateful he'd noticed and was offering me a lifeline, but it was a tricky one: Friday was Dr Bruno's Craniofacial Surgery clinic, which was often busy. I didn't want to let him down, or make life hard for Caleb and Bernadette. Plus, he had given me that publication opportunity.

I ended up reluctantly taking the Friday off. I was due to work twelve days in a row from the following Monday so it seemed the only sensible thing to do. I was worried as I typed the email informing Dr Bruno and the team. I think they probably did feel let down, though they never said anything. I went back to my apartment on the Thursday night feeling guilty, but so desperate for rest. What a conundrum this life was. I was sad my time at the hospital was about to end. It had been one of my favourite terms as a doctor – I loved working with children, the consultant surgeons were supportive, and the work was rewarding. But despite an environment that was much more supportive than those I'd been used to, in some ways those last weeks showed me that, even then, in Surgery it was every person for themselves. It seemed we were all so run down by the system that, in the end, few of us had the reserves to help another out.

Nevertheless, I felt really optimistic about the year ahead. Twenty-eighteen was going to be my year – I could feel it flowing through me. I believed in willing things to happen. I believed in positive thinking, in visualising success. I could picture myself being accepted into the Program. I had got so close to selection in previous years. Surely 2018 would be my time.

PART 4

Teacher

30

This is going to be my year

2018, *New South Wales*

I had a steep mountain to climb. Only the highest in Australia: Mount Kosciuszko.

It was the first week of January and I had signed up for a triathlon camp. We had cycled from Jindabyne to Thredbo, and then started the climb up Kosciuszko. It was literally an uphill struggle. I hadn't noticed much weight gain during my term at the Children's Hospital, but it was becoming clear to me that I was less fit, and heavier, than I had been in previous years. I was hating every second of the ride, and feeling frustrated and hopeless up the hill. Usually, I pushed myself along with positive self-talk, but I had no such compassion for myself this time. There was no riding, just internal deriding.

After a while I gave up and hopped into the support car for the ride of shame up the hill. Just over a year ago I was fit enough to run a marathon. No matter how stressed I was in previous years, I'd almost always managed to balance work with exercise. I told myself that I really needed to get back on track. This was not acceptable.

Hayden, the coach, came up to me later. 'It's all in the mind,' he said. *Not if you're unfit*, I thought to myself. I was embarrassed to be there. But I needed to do it because it was going to help me for another ride I had signed up to for the Children's Hospital Burns Unit. It was a charity ride organised by Fire and Rescue NSW, in which firefighters would be riding from Wagga Wagga to Sydney over four days in March. *C'mon, Yumiko, this is good training*.

The next day I was up early for a time trial ascending Kosciuszko to Charlotte Pass. I was dreading it and contemplated sitting it out, but I pulled up my big girl socks and showed up. Within 10 kilometres, the others started to take over. 'Hello!' 'Looking good!' 'Keep going!' 'Nice work!' they cheered as they cycled past me, pushing themselves up the hill. I replied with a huff here and a grunt there. No matter how hard it was, I told myself that I was not going to jump into the car today. I didn't care if I was nearly stationary on the steepest parts of the course, I wasn't going to stop moving my legs. *Charlotte Pass – I'm coming to get you*. I was as determined as the march flies that clawed through my shorts.

I knew the end was near when I spotted some cars parked along the road. At the top of the last little incline I saw my triathlon group. I'd made it! I was so glad I hadn't given up. I knew that this was going to be symbolic for the rest of my year.

My new term as a plastic surgery registrar started a few weeks later, in south-west Sydney. I was going to be working with accredited registrar Amos in the hospital's Plastics department. A week before I started, Amos emailed me the on-call roster, apparently a copy-and-paste of the previous term's. Ten days a fortnight for me; four for Amos. I'd also be covering Ear, Nose and Throat surgery at the hospital for eight of those days, despite having close to no experience in it.

I messaged the registrar who had done the job before me to confirm that this was really the deal. It was. Aware of the importance of this term in the annual selection process for the Program, I decided I'd just have to suck it up. The roster was a fait accompli. I had a look at the handover document, which outlined who I'd be working with. The surgeons included Dr Sansevieria, whom I'd heard of through Dr Whiteley, and Dr Nepenthes, whom I needed to impress. He had connections with the selection panel for the Program, wielding enormous power. It was a bit odd to me that he'd have a public hospital appointment in the south-west, when he lived in a far wealthier area, beside a glittering, postcard-worthy beach, but it turned out he'd had a humble upbringing. Perhaps working here was his way of giving back to communities like the one that had raised him. I'd also be working with an ENT surgeon, Dr Demir, and an unaccredited ENT registrar called Simon.

On my first day, I met the juniors on my team. My resident, Kevin, was full of energy and was keen on surgery – Urology in particular. We also had a medical student, Thea, who was doing a rotation in Plastic Surgery. She wanted to be a GP when she finished medical school. Even though surgery was not her *raison d'être*, she still showed up early every day, and came with me to every operation. She was one of those students who wanted to make the most of every opportunity available. They were both fantastic. I couldn't have asked for lovelier helpers. I felt positive about the term ahead; having a good team made such a difference.

After our first ward round together, I ordered some coffees and banana bread via a phone app, then ducked into the bathrooms near Emergency while Kevin went to collect our morning snack. As I walked in, I stalled. The lighting was funny and disorientating. I turned the light switch off and back on again, but it was still too dark to see properly. Maybe it was because I'd just walked through Emergency, which was very brightly lit. It was a weird UV light, like I'd just walked into a spin studio. I shrugged it off and went into a cubicle, where I noticed a yellow sharps bin pinned to the wall. Ah. Blue lights so that people don't shoot up in the toilets. Got it. I wasn't a prude, but it still shocked me a little. I'd treated many patients who were current or ex-intravenous drug users, but I'd never worked anywhere with blue lights in the toilets. It made me wonder whether I'd have to deal with ice rage on this new job.

The Plastic Surgery consultants were pleased with my previous experience in hand surgery – it meant they could take Amos over to the private hospital to help them with their major cases while I manned the fort. It felt good to know that they trusted my operative skills and ability to manage the patients on my own; however, immediately I was on the back foot because my department was severely under-resourced. Plastic surgery dressings are sometimes complex and time-consuming, which make nurses an essential part of Plastics clinics. We had no nurse for our clinic. We literally didn't even have a Band-Aid solution.

Our staffing issues didn't stop there. We didn't have any hand therapists, who provide physiotherapy before and after surgery. They help manage pain. They make splints. The catchment area for the hospital was not a wealthy area of Sydney. I was concerned that some patients would not be able to afford a private hand therapist. How could we be a public health service operating on people's hands and not offer them the routine post-operative care they need? These were all things that I felt were unacceptable, but the unit consultants were already well aware of the shortages. They reassured me that all were on their 'wish list' of things for the unit, which I suspected hadn't changed since 1999. The area had experienced huge population growth over the last couple of decades and was one of the busiest hospitals in New South Wales. Yet it struggled with funding and resources.

By the second week, I'd started to sleep over at the hospital because the days were long and I didn't feel safe enough to drive home to the North Shore. My exercise routine had almost overnight slipped away because there weren't any gyms near work. I was far too busy to exercise, in any case. I knew I must be gaining weight with every order of hot chips I had at the hospital café, but I was in survival mode – when I was constantly rushing from A to B I needed to eat quickly. I wasn't at home enough to cook, so I stocked the office cupboard with emergency snacks.

When March came around, I wasn't in a great physical condition for the charity cycle. On the day I was due to ride, I made my way to Bowral to join the firefighters for the last 100 kilometres. Within my first few pedal strokes, I knew I was in trouble. My brain was so fatigued that at every traffic light I couldn't get my cleats to click back into my pedals.

I felt totally uncoordinated. I was a lot slower than the rest of the group and at the end, as we were preparing to cycle into the hospital, I fell off my bike during a momentary lapse of concentration. How embarrassing! But also it was frightening that my fatigue was affecting me that much.

The day after the ride, Kevin told me that he'd be taking an allocated day off the following Tuesday. I told him that was fine, and we agreed we'd make sure there was a replacement for him. However, after a few days a reliever still hadn't been organised, so we went to see the Junior Medical Officer manager, who was in charge of rostering.

'I understand Kevin's been given a day off next Tuesday. Which resident will be covering for him, please?' I asked her.

'I don't think there will be anyone,' she answered.

'So who's going to be covering the wards then?' I asked.

'You will,' she said bluntly.

I could feel my heart pounding. This was ridiculous. I knew it would be impossible for me to carry the JMO pager and do paperwork on the ward, as well as complete all my registrar responsibilities. 'What if I'm operating? I can't attend to emergencies on the ward if I'm in the middle of an operation.' I was coming out in cold sweats as I imagined having to run around the ward with two pagers bleeping from my waist, doing tasks like putting in intravenous cannulas, while taking referrals from the Emergency Department. Even worse, if I were to be operating on a patient, the pagers would be sitting by the computer in the operating theatre, unanswered, with irate people on the other end waiting for me to return their page.

'Sorry, I'm not in charge of allocations,' said the JMO manager.

'Yumiko, it's okay, I won't take my ADO,' reassured Kevin.

'No, no. You're entitled to your ADO. I can't take that away from you.' But my heart was sinking just imagining the potential chaos next Tuesday might bring.

'Well, maybe I can take it on another day,' suggested Kevin.

'Could you?'

'Yeah. I haven't planned anything for next Tuesday anyway.'

'Are you sure, Kevin?'

'Yeah, I'm sure.'

I felt bad that Kevin's day off had been torpedoed, but so grateful to him. In this dog-eat-dog world it gave me enormous relief that there were people like Kevin who were willing to help a colleague out. Crisis averted.

31

Cancel culture

2018, Sydney

Friday afternoons were the worst time to book operations. It took only a few weeks of being at the hospital to realise how inefficient the theatre was, especially on weekends. If the surgery didn't happen on the Friday, there was a good chance the patient would not be operated on until Monday.

Week three, and on the Friday a man named Aram in his late twenties was referred to me, having injured his thumb after losing a fight with some heavy furniture. He had lost quite a lot of flesh, so he needed a flap of skin to cover the wound. It was already 4 pm and I had a familiar, uneasy feeling in my stomach. I pressed 'play' for my pre-recorded spiel: 'I have booked your operation, and hope to get it done today. However, if a patient comes in with a serious condition and needs more urgent surgery, we may be delayed. If we are unlucky, we may be deferred until Monday.' I also had to remind Aram that he was unable to eat or drink anything until the operation was completed: after eating, you can't be operated on for six hours, otherwise there's a risk of aspirating food into your lungs when you're under a general anaesthetic.

Beep. A page from the operating theatre. I rang back, and to my astonishment they were ready for me. Maybe luck was on my side today. I called Kevin and told him that he and Thea should go home.

'You sure? Do you need any help in theatre?'

'I'm good. Thanks for your hard work this week,' I said. Kevin and Thea were always willing to stay and help, they were good like that, but there was no way I was making them hang back on a Friday afternoon. I rushed to the surgery via the café, knowing I might not get a chance to buy dinner later, and scoffed down a falafel wrap as I walked up the stairs to the operating theatre. My mother would be appalled. Eating while walking is considered rude in Japan, and I probably ate on the go more frequently than I did at a table.

Aram was visiting from Lebanon and had overseas insurance. Surgeons are usually interested in such cases because they can charge a handsome fee to the insurance company, but the consultants whose public work was in this hospital tended to feel that the drive wasn't worth it for them. Most of them lived near the coast and it would take them close to two hours to come this way in peak-hour traffic. I called Dr Nepenthes to inform him of the case. As expected, he was happy for me to proceed on my own.

I was in a good mood. For once, I could get my surgery done. I went to the change rooms to get into my blue scrubs and greeted the anaesthetist and nurses. We enjoyed a bit of chit-chat as I started preparing for the case. I was planning on repairing Aram's amputated thumb with a flap and I had a checklist in my head: arm tourniquet – check. Arm table – check. Sutures – check. Dressings – check. Plaster trolley – check. We were good to go. All we needed was the patient. Restlessly, I walked over to the pre-operative area to help collect him. I wanted to get things rolling before we got cancelled by an Emergency Caesarean section, which was a constant threat.

In front of the operating theatre, I saw Aram, who smiled and waved. The administrative clerk, Sandra, was standing nearby.

'Ah! Plastics. I need to talk to you,' she said.

'Oh, I'm about to do an operation,' I said.

'Yes, it's about that,' said Sandra. 'We can't go ahead because we can't confirm the patient's insurance status.'

'His uncle said that his overseas insurance covers him,' I said.

'We can't go on his word. We need the paperwork from his insurance company,' she explained. 'They're not picking up their phones, but I'll keep trying.'

Helen, the nurse in charge, joined us. 'We're going to have to let another team go first,' she said. 'You can go after them, I promise.'

I couldn't believe it. The one time I thought I'd get an operation done during normal daylight hours, I was delayed due to paperwork.

I went to the surgical registrars' office to do some other work. Dr Bruno had sent me an email with changes to the article we were writing on breast cancer reconstruction. I opened the document with his annotations, and started addressing each comment one by one, but after an hour I couldn't concentrate on the paper anymore, so I returned to the operating theatre to see if any progress had been made with the insurance company.

'I was just about to call you,' said Sandra.

'Great, are we going ahead?' I asked optimistically.

'No, their office has closed for the day,' she said. 'But they're open on Saturdays. I'll get the weekend clerk to ring them first thing in the morning.'

Dreading the conversation with Aram, I went to find him on the ward. He was already eating his dinner, pre-empting my apology.

When I was working at the Children's Hospital, weekends off were a time for activities like yoga, running, coastal walks, bike rides and café brunches with friends. These days I spent the weekends either working, or slumped in my apartment recovering from my twelve-day fortnight. This weekend I was at the hospital, and on the Saturday morning a new patient was referred to me. An elderly gentleman by the name of Mr Pilea had a finger infection. It was initially lanced by his GP, but it had come back more swollen and red.

I treated Mr Pilea in the Emergency Department. A lot of pus came out of his finger so I irrigated the wound with copious amounts of antiseptic and explained that it was possible we might have to do an operation if the infection didn't improve, but for now the plan was for intravenous antibiotics and daily dressings.

By mid-morning the administrative staff had been able to get in touch with Aram's insurance company, who had confirmed that the surgery would be covered under his policy.

He was placed back in the queue for surgery. In the meantime I was getting phone calls about all sorts of things, from ENT stuff to Plastics. I remained anxious covering ENT because of my lack of experience. I prided myself in the way I conducted my consultations and was frankly terrified of the prospect of being asked something I knew nothing about: I didn't want to come across to any patient as an idiot, and I certainly didn't want to make any mistakes in my recommendations or treatment.

In the afternoon I was called about a little boy, Joe, who'd had his tonsils out a few days prior by Dr Demir in his capacity as a private surgeon. Joe was sore and unable to eat. I had a look in his throat and everything looked fine, but I admitted him so that we could get better control of his pain and look after him until he was comfortably able to swallow some food. He was a private patient so I thought I'd better inform Dr Demir. When I rang him, his brusque response was 'I'm not on call.'

'Yes, I know. I'm sorry to bother you, but this is about a private patient,' I said. 'Joe was on your list a few days ago for a tonsillectomy and I've admitted him for pain relief.'

'Don't call me when I'm not on call,' he said, and hung up the phone.

I was bewildered by the interaction. Not only was I stunned by how rude he was, but the more concerning thing was that it appeared he felt no duty of care towards his patient. He'd operated on this little boy – wasn't he concerned about how his patient was doing post-operatively? I walked back to the registrars' office to work on my article, which I really needed to send back to Dr Bruno. Before I knew it, it was 10 pm and I had the usual sinking feeling in my gut. As a general rule, operating theatres did not run late at night unless it was urgent, because night shift staff were sparse. Time to cancel Aram.

On the Sunday ward round, a crowd of men – I assumed relatives – stood around Aram. They were seething. One of them – his uncle, I later found out – walked up to me, standing very close to my face. He was a physically intimidating, muscular man, who towered over me.

'Why was Aram cancelled again?' he screamed. 'How can you make him starve all fucking day and just cancel him?' The other patients in the cubicle looked awkwardly away.

'I'm sorry,' I said, taking a step back. 'Unfortunately, there were a lot of urgent cases yesterday.' At that point, the nurse in charge entered the cubicle to back me up.

'Sir, please, it's not the doctor's fault,' she said.

'This is fucked up,' he said, and stormed out of the ward.

I exhaled. The nurse put her hand on my shoulder, looking sorry for me.

I hurried to the operating theatre to see what was happening and was reassured that Aram would be first on the list and I would be called straightaway. In the other wards I finished the rest of my morning round, then ordered a coffee to get me fuelled up. With cup in hand, I walked back to the operating theatre to see if Aram was there yet.

'Ah, Yumiko!' called out the nurse in charge, Asha. She was heavily pregnant, only a week away from taking maternity leave.

'Morning, Asha,' I said. 'Are you in charge today?'

'Yes.'

'Am I still going first?' I asked.

'Yes, you are,' she said. 'But there's an issue. We have an electricity outage.'

'Oh, that's okay. I can operate in the dark, no worries,' I joked.

'I'm so sorry, I know this patient has been cancelled a few times.'

'Yeah, the uncle was not very happy with me this morning. He was kind of aggressive, actually,' I said.

'The maintenance staff are on to it,' she said. 'I'll call you as soon as we're ready for you.'

'Okay, thanks. I won't be far. I'll just be in my office so I can come at five minutes' notice,' I said. The lack of electricity was absurd to me, it felt like I was dreaming. I was so tired that I easily could have been.

I went off to the surgical registrars' office and checked my emails. Dr Bruno had sent back my article with a few changes, and wanted to use an image he'd found in another article. Every time I sent something back, I seemed to get even more changes, but I trusted Dr Bruno. He had a very high standard when it came to research articles. I managed to track down the image he wanted and wrote to the corresponding author, who was based in the UK. There was nothing more I could do to move things forward – I just had to wait for her reply. It felt like my life. Always waiting. Waiting for permission to use this image, waiting for operating time, waiting to get selected on to the Program. When would I feel like I was no longer waiting, and just living?

A few hours later I was finally called to the operating theatre. Aram was in the anaesthetic bay, ready to be wheeled in.

'Can I go to the bathroom?' he asked.

Off he and the anaesthetic nurse went as she escorted him to the toilet.

Meanwhile, I set up in the operating room. Having ticked off everything on my checklist, I was ready to go.

The phone rang and the anaesthetist, Gerald, picked up. He covered the phone to speak to me and Asha.

'It's Obstetrics,' he said. 'Caesar.'

'What category is it?' Asha asked.

'Category three,' he said.

What a relief. That meant they could go after me.

'Plastics is doing a quick case now, and then we'll do your Caesar,' he said down the phone. 'How long will your case be?' he asked me.

'About an hour,' I replied. Gerald relayed that information on.

'They're making it category two,' he said.

'Wait, *what?*' I felt my ears starting to get hot. 'They can't just change the category so that they can go before me!'

'We have to let them go first,' said Asha.

'No,' I said. 'That's so unfair. They only changed the category because Gerald told them they have to wait an hour.'

'I know, but on paper it says they've booked a category two Caesarean section,' said Asha. 'If anything happens to the baby, it's my fault.'

I looked at Asha's pregnant belly and I knew that I couldn't argue.

'This is ridiculous,' I said, fuming. 'If the patient hadn't gone to the toilet he'd be asleep on the operating table and we'd have started by now.'

I walked out of the operating theatre to find Aram's family waiting outside.

'Oh!' yelled out Aram's uncle. 'How'd it go, doc?'

I couldn't even look at him, I was so upset. How was I supposed to explain that Aram had been cancelled for a third time? Fortuitously, my phone rang, so I gestured to him that I needed to pick up.

'Hello? Yumiko speaking,' I answered, hot-footing it towards my office.

I walked inside, closed the door and burst into tears. I was so tired and frustrated. It was my eighth day in a row of doing a twenty-four-hour on-call shift. I just couldn't believe the temerity of those obstetricians to manipulate clinical triage categories to suit themselves. *Aram, you had all day to go to the toilet!*

Aram ended up being another 'Friday to Monday' patient, who gets booked on the Friday, waits all weekend and doesn't get his operation until the Monday.

32

Burning the midnight oil

2018, Sydney

Dr Nepenthes was the on-call consultant again. He was ringing to let me know that he was sending a private patient to the Emergency Department: a seven-year-old boy who'd lost the tip of his finger after getting it caught trampolining.

The little boy and his mother arrived, his mother carrying a Ziploc bag containing the end of his pinky. This case was time-critical but Obstetrics were doing yet another emergency Caesarean section so I wouldn't get any theatre time for a couple of hours. I explained the situation to the boy's mother and spent about twenty minutes assessing her son, explaining the surgery, the risks and potential complications. When I'd finished she said, 'Nurse, when do we get to see the doctor?'

'Er. I am the doctor,' I said, feeling a little awkward and, frankly, flummoxed. I was fairly sure that I had introduced myself as Yumiko, 'the doctor', when I'd approached them.

Then again, it wasn't the first time that I had been mistaken for a nurse or a medical student. Did patients honestly think I wasn't old enough to be a doctor? I was now thirty, in my eighth year of working and the idea of still having to prove my competence was more and more disheartening. When patients decide you don't look old enough, it's as though they lack confidence in your care. 'Asians don't raisin,' they say. Not a single wrinkle inhabited my face, but sometimes I wished there were a frown line or two to represent the years I'd spent concentrating on a textbook, or focusing on an operation.

Or maybe it wasn't my age this time. When I looked up at that proverbial ceiling, was it made from bamboo or glass? Perhaps a hybrid of both. Despite the viral hashtag #ILookLikeASurgeon in 2015, women still had to work a lot harder than men to be regarded as legitimate surgeons. Being an Asian female made it even worse. With the Philippines being the biggest exporter of nurses globally, I'd worked with a lot of Filipino nurses over the past eight years. I wondered whether that made it easy for people to assume I was a nurse? All of these things crossed my mind every time I got called 'nurse' or 'student'. It was tiring.

It was nearly 9 pm when I eventually got to operate on the boy. I put on my loupes and carefully sutured back the tip of his finger, including his nail bed, using sutures that are finer than eyelashes. The operation itself was short – a composite graft takes less than ten minutes to do – but we had waited all evening.

As I changed out of scrubs and back into my 'civvy' clothes, I got a phone call from the Emergency Department about a man who'd cut three of his fingers while slicing some vegetables:

after he was done with the cutting, he'd planted the knife into the wooden chopping board and his fingers slid on the blade. Since I was already in the hospital, I decided to see him on my way out. I was a one-woman band. If I didn't see him then, it was an extra patient for me in the morning. No one would be taking over. It was just me.

After assessing him, it was clear a long operation lay ahead. His fingers flopped off his hand like a ragdoll – he'd obviously cut through his tendons. All three fingers had patches of numbness, and one was pale. I added them up in my head: four tendons, a few nerves, at least, and maybe an artery or two. Plus, it was his dominant hand and he was a manual labourer.

I knew I had to inform Dr Nepenthes of the case but I was reluctant to call him. It was late at night and he was probably asleep. Also he and I had a big case to do the next day – a woman with breast cancer who would need both breasts reconstructed using a large free flap from her abdomen. I held the phone to my ear and the ring tone gnawed at my eardrums a few times before he picked up.

'You're good at micro, aren't you? You'll be fine. See you tomorrow,' he said, and hung up the phone. Solo again. I let out a noise, something between a sigh and a yawn. It echoed in the empty entrance chamber of the hospital. I returned to the operating theatre to change back into scrubs.

'I have an urgent case – a man with a hand injury with concerns about the circulation to one of his fingers,' I explained to the anaesthetist and nurse in charge, who had come on for the night shift. While we waited for the patient to be admitted and sent up to the operating theatre from Emergency, the anaesthetist shared a bit of his dinner with me. His wife had packed him some grilled vegetables and halloumi. Moments like these made me wish I had a wife, too – this was the healthiest and most delicious meal I'd eaten for days. I'd heard an aphorism that if you start life as a registrar single, you'll remain single. There's no time to foster relationships, not even the one you have with yourself; to be mindful of your own needs, develop self-awareness and be compassionate towards yourself. I wasn't even able to prioritise basic self-care like food and sleep. I was probably lonely, as well, but I was too busy to dwell on that. I helped myself to a piece of grilled eggplant and drank some tea to perk myself up.

'Isn't your boss coming in for a big case like this?' the anaesthetist asked. I shook my head. I couldn't remember the last time I'd seen a boss. Even so, I was determined to do a good job. This was a complex operation and this man's livelihood depended on it. No pressure.

My eyes were sore, but as soon as they peered down the microscope, they focused and I slipped into autopilot mode. I gently placed the man's hand into a lead hand, which held each finger back, holding them still. As I'd predicted from my assessment, the knife had cut through several tendons. The end of one tendon had retracted into the palm, so I went on a little fishing expedition to retrieve it. It really was like trying to take control of a live fish because the muscles in the forearm kept pulling the tendon back into the palm. Moments like these reminded me that having Dr Nepenthes there – or anyone – would have made life a lot easier. Nevertheless, I persisted. After repairing all of the tendons, it was time to repair the nerves that lay on either side of them. By this stage I was fatigued and my eyes felt like they'd been sandpapered. Even when I finished all the repairs inside the fingers, I still had to sew up the skin on each finger. There were about fifteen small stitches in each, not that I would have counted them but for the patients, who always asked, 'How many stitches?' And then I put the dressings on and made a plaster to protect the hand.

It took me four hours, but I was proud of the microsurgery I'd performed, especially without another surgeon who would usually be present for any kind of microsurgical procedure. Even though I was drained, I knew that I could not have done any better for this patient, and that gave me a deep sense of satisfaction. I walked into the recovery ward to ask a nurse for a key to the staff overnight rooms.

'No, we can't give you the keys. They're only for night-shift staff.'

I was too tired to argue. I drew the blue paper curtains to cordon off a small section of Recovery to myself, took a shower in the theatre changerooms, turned my undies inside out, and put on some fresh scrubs to wear as pyjamas. By the time I had finished writing my operation report, it was 4 am. I tried to fall sleep to the sound of machines beeping and the night-shift nurses chatting. Two hours later the morning-shift nurses turned on the blindingly white lights. I bee-lined to the café and waited for it to open at 6.30, aching for a coffee. I would need it – the breast reconstruction was going to take all day.

After the ward round I went to Outpatients to check up on Mr Pilea, my elderly patient with the finger infection. He had sort of become my social life. Mr Pilea was the only person I saw regularly, and he was always very pleasant and grateful for my care. Then I made my way to the operating theatre to see Dr Nepenthes and Dr Sansevieria.

'Was I dreaming or did you call me last night?' asked Dr Nepenthes.

'I did,' I replied. 'It ended up being four tendons and two nerves. Thankfully, the arteries were intact.'

'You legend,' he said, patting me on the back. He looked at Dr Sansevieria. 'How good is it that the registrars this term can do tendons?'

'We're very lucky,' she said.

Later that morning, I asked Dr Sansevieria if I could take a break. I told her that I'd only had two hours of sleep.

'I remember doing those sorts of hours as a registrar,' she said. 'It's good for you, you'll be fine.'

That weekend, I was on call again. I was covering ENT, so I received a handover from Simon, who told me that Dr Demir was the consultant on call. I felt my heart sink. 'He was very short with me on the phone once. I'm not sure that he likes me,' I said.

'Yeah, he always groans when I tell him you're on call,' said Simon. 'You know what bosses are like, especially on the weekends. They don't want to be bothered.'

It irked me – consultant surgeons who didn't want to do their jobs. Why bother even having a public hospital appointment? Did it give them more credibility if they could write on their websites that they were training younger surgeons? It wasn't my fault that the hospital made me cover ENT. As junior doctors we couldn't be expected to know everything – there were always going to be firsts. What I really needed was for Dr Demir to be understanding and supportive, not for him to groan whenever I was on call with him.

On the Saturday morning, I was referred a middle-aged man with a fishbone stuck in his throat. I dreaded needing to call in Dr Demir but I knew I'd have to. I told the patient that I'd contact the consultant, but that he might be about an hour away.

'Can't you get it out, doc?' the patient asked.

'I'm usually a Plastic Surgery doctor; I'm just covering Ear, Nose and Throat,' I explained. 'It's been several years since I've used a scope down someone's nose.'

'Can you give it a go? Please?' he asked. 'I'm desperate for this bone to be out, it's killing me.'

'I can, but there's a chance I might still have to call the consultant if I'm not able to retrieve it,' I explained.

I skipped up the stairs two at a time to the operating theatres to get the nasendoscope. I already felt bad enough for the guy, I wasn't going to make him wait longer than he needed to. The pressure was on. I was up for the challenge, mainly because I didn't want to ring Dr Demir and give him more reasons to groan. I remembered my friend Frank teaching me how to use a nasendoscope in 2013 when I was a resident in Melbourne. I'd practised on my colleague Noah.

Back in the cubicle, I sprayed some anaesthetic into the man's nose and throat. I was lucky that he wasn't squeamish and sat still as I navigated the flimsy tube up his nose, and down the back of his throat. It didn't take long for me to spot the offending bone, a surprisingly small one, lying in an area called the piriform fossa. It was amazing how something so small could cause such a lot of discomfort.

Spotting it was one thing, trying to grab it was another. With one hand I held the scope and with the other a pair of forceps. I tussled with the bone for a while, trying not to lose my patience. I was determined to fetch that damn bone.

'Got it!' I announced in triumph, as I pulled it out.

'Oh, thank god!' exclaimed the patient. I don't know who was happier – him or me.

'Can I keep it?' he asked.

'Sure.' I placed the bone into his palm.

'Wow, tiny, hey?' he said, staring at it.

It was exhilarating. I had forgotten the joys of being a trainee surgeon. I'd forgotten how exciting it was to practise a new skill and be able to make a patient happy. Using a nasendoscope was the best thing to have happened all year, as sad as that sounds. Also, I hadn't had to call Dr Demir. I could just imagine his resentment at being asked to come in for a fishbone!

My Sunday-night ritual was to throw out fresh produce from my fridge because I was barely at home to cook, but the following evening I got home at a reasonable time so I decided I'd better not waste the vegetables I'd bought earlier in the week. I took the carrot and zucchini out of the fridge and gave them a quick rinse. They'd gone a bit soft but I chopped them all up and threw them into the frying pan. As I did so, the water I'd washed them in fought with the hot oil in the pan, causing an explosive splash, which landed on my right hand. *Fuck.* I rushed to the kitchen sink and started running cold water over my hand.

In the meantime, the vegetables turned black and stuck to my old pan like limpets to a rock. Having just done a six-month rotation treating children's burns, I knew better than to stop the cold water, but who really has time to stand there for twenty minutes? I ignored my own medical advice and turned off the tap. Doctors make the worst patients. I threw out my vegetables, which would've been thrown out anyway, and sighed. *So, this is what happens when I try to be good and cook a meal at home, eh?*

Before I could feel too sorry for myself, my phone rang.

'Hello, is that Plastics?'

'Yes, it is,' I replied.

'I have a category two,' said the Emergency registrar.

'What do you mean by that?' I asked.

'It's limb-threatening,' she said. 'This man has a partial amputation through his thumb joint.'

'Okay, I'll come in,' I said, as I grabbed my keys off the kitchen counter. I had a quick look at the stove to make sure I'd turned it off, before taking the lift down to the car park. As I grabbed the steering wheel, I could see the burn on the back of my hand. It looked nasty and it stung for the whole drive to the hospital.

When I arrived in the Emergency Department I scanned the room for a 'category two'. *Where is the man with his thumb falling off?* I eventually found a nurse who helped me to locate the patient – a man in his forties wearing hi-vis. He had a wound just underneath his thumbnail, which was nowhere near his joint. I tried to keep it professional and hide my annoyance at the registrar who'd called me in.

I put on some gloves to hide the burn on my hand. 'I want to reassure you that this will heal,' I told him. 'I'm going to clean this wound and put a dressing on it.'

'Oh, the other lady said I needed surgery,' he said.

I really wished Emergency doctors wouldn't tell patients that they need or don't need surgery.

'No,' I said. 'Thankfully, you don't. It's a shallow wound and the skin in this area heals very well because it has a good blood supply.'

On my way out, I grabbed a dressing to put on my burn. At the exit, I bumped into the urology registrar, Peter. If anyone in the hospital understood my life, it would be him. Pete had to manage so much on-call because his co-registrar was on indefinite family leave of some sort.

'You got called in too?' I asked.

'Yeah, a torsion,' he replied.

'Fair enough,' I said with a sympathetic smile. At least that's a true emergency, I thought. Mine was not. I had trusted the Emergency registrar's assessment and description of the injury. Words like 'category two', 'partial amputation' and 'limb-threatening' had brought me straight to the hospital. I wondered whether Pete would see a patient with a real testicular torsion or whether that also might be fake news.

As I got to my car my stomach growled. I looked at the clock: 10.30 pm. At that time of night, a drive-through meal was my only choice. I was ravenous and craved something fatty to fill me up. Thankfully there were hardly any cars on the road so it didn't take me long to find something. I substituted a soft drink with water to make myself feel better about ordering junk food. I placed my meal on the passenger seat and realised it had been a while since I'd had anyone on that seat. It was only in these quiet moments that I was reminded that not only did there seem no hope of finding a boyfriend when I was working these hours, but I had no family in Australia. I thought about my parents and my sisters. I hadn't called to ask how Hajime was going with his lymphoma. *What a bad daughter I am.* I made a mental note to phone them during the week.

The next morning, I told Dr Sansevieria about the patient I got called in for. 'You should have asked them to text you a photo,' she said.

Kevin was a bit more sympathetic. 'Damn, that's annoying,' he said.

'Yeah, but I'm glad for the patient that it was nothing serious,' I said. 'He thought there was *thumb*-thing wrong.'

'Oh Yumiko, that's a terrible pun!' he said, before noticing the burn on my hand. It was a second-degree burn and looked worse than it had last night.

'What happened?'

'My frying pan exploded,' I laughed as we started our ward round.

'It looks sore!'

'Yeah, it does still sting a little,' I replied.

'Are you going to be able to operate?'

'I'll just stick a Tegaderm over it,' I said matter-of-factly, before I realised that Kevin had just given me an idea. Whenever we have small wounds, we cover them with a waterproof dressing that still allows us to wash our hands and perform surgery. *What if I injured myself so that I couldn't scrub for surgery anymore?* Maybe *then* I wouldn't have to do operations in the middle of the night on my own, and maybe they'd get done by Amos, or the consultants, who would have to make themselves available for once.

It scared me a little – were things so bad now that I was thinking of hurting myself?

33

Shit hits the fan

2018, Sydney

I continued to check up on Mr Pilea, whose finger infection was improving but still needing daily care, even when I wasn't working. Amos refused to do his dressings when he was on call on the weekends. He claimed it was a nurse's job. 'But we don't have any nurses,' I pointed out. That didn't persuade him to help out, and I didn't know whether he'd do a good enough job with the dressings, anyhow. Plus, I'd looked after Mr Pilea's finger infection for several weeks now, I knew what he needed and it was nice for the same person to monitor the wound for continuity of care. So I'd come in on weekends to review Mr Pilea's finger and change his dressings, and then go home.

My own wound wasn't looking too good. I knew none of the consultant surgeons I worked with now would care, but I knew someone who would – Uncle Phil. I had kept in touch with him so I decided to take a photo of my burn to send him. It had blistered and started to peel off, showing a raw red bit in the middle. He replied straight away. 'Looks painful! I'm sorry for you.' At least someone was kind. Thank you, Uncle Phil.

On Monday, after Amos had been on call at the weekend, he handed me over a patient to operate on. The patient had come in on Sunday afternoon and Amos had told her not to worry about staying 'nil by mouth' because the operating theatre was too busy for the surgery to take place any time soon. By letting the patient eat, Amos was able to delay her to Monday because of the rule that you can't have surgery within six hours of eating. Unfortunately for Amos, the patient was a family friend of Dr Nepenthes, and Dr Nepenthes decided to call the operating theatre, only to find that it was, in fact, not busy at all. As though I didn't already have enough going on, my colleague was increasing my workload behind my back. Even though I'd learned to put up with these sorts of games, part of me was glad that certain incidents such as this one got back to the consultants. At least they knew some of what was happening at ground level, even if they didn't know exactly how hard I was working every day, because *they* changed over every day.

The thought of hurting myself had, initially, been a fleeting one, but today it started to pervade my thoughts. I had done on-call work plenty of times, and had worked long days, but I was finding the work here different. I was on call almost continually. That meant I was in a constant state of mental unrest. My body was a machine on stand-by at all times. It's not the same as completely switching off; more like sleeping with one eye open. Even when I did get alternate weekends off, I didn't feel refreshed.

And now all I could think about in my spare moments was how I could injure my hands. I had to injure them enough so that I couldn't do any operations, but not so much that I'd have a permanent injury and lose my career. *Maybe I need to burn myself more significantly* . . . But I didn't want to require a skin graft. That's more hassle than it's worth. *Maybe I could punch a wall and break my hand?* Again, not worth it if I ended up needing an operation. *What if I stab myself somewhere that isn't too important in the palm?* Through my knowledge of hand anatomy I knew to avoid certain areas because I could potentially damage nerves, arteries, and tendons . . . but there were parts of the palm that were mostly muscle. Maybe I could give one of them a stab.

The next time I was in the Emergency Department treating a patient, I found myself staring at the disposable scalpels. I pulled myself up. What was I *doing*? This wasn't normal.

'Are you all right there?' a nurse asked.

'Yeah, I'm fine, sorry. Just in a bit of a daydream!' I forced a laugh.

'Are you admitting that patient?'

'Yes, yes, I am,' I said, and completed the paperwork.

I glanced again at the scalpels. *There's no way I would actually do it*, I told myself; the thoughts in my head were just hypothetical.

That night, I finally found some time to FaceTime my father. Hajime's last PET scan showed that his lymphoma had spread, and he would be starting chemotherapy with a relatively new drug regimen that I hadn't heard of in medical school. I could see that Dad wasn't taking care of himself. He was usually well-groomed but now he had an unkempt beard and his hair hadn't been as long since his hippie days in the seventies.

'You look like you're due for a haircut, Dad,' I pointed out.

'What's the point in cutting my hair? I'm going to lose it when I go through chemo anyway,' he replied nonchalantly. Fair enough. I had no rebuttal for that.

'I'll try to get some annual leave to come and visit you when you start your chemo,' I said, knowing that this might not happen. As soon as I hung up, I wrote an email to Dr Sansevieria with my request. I desperately wanted to go to Japan to see my family. I knew that as the only medical person in my family, they would find my presence reassuring. So I was nervous about what her response might be – doctors had their leave requests rejected all the time. There was even a plastic surgeon who famously did a ward round on the morning of her own wedding!

The next morning I went to see the JMO manager, to fill out a leave-request form. I also handed in my timesheet. By then, in my first month of working, I'd accumulated a hundred hours of overtime. The manager was quick to handball the responsibility to Dr Sansevieria: 'I don't do your roster, you need to talk to your own department,' she said.

It was late March and I was miserable, truly exhausted. I was driving to work one morning when I felt something warm and wet in my pants. Wait. Could it be? I kept going for another minute, wondering what the hell to do. Do I keep driving or have I actually lost faecal continence? I pulled over and gingerly lifted up my skirt. Shit. Literal shit. It was horrifying. But I had no time to feel sorry for myself. I needed to get to work. It felt like I was in a bad dream. It was, of course, a day I was wearing beautiful satin and lace undies.

I got out of the car, hid behind the passenger door and took off my undies. They were completely soiled. My car was still strewn with beach towels from the last time I'd managed to make it to the beach, which must have been a few months previously. I took the one covered in the least amount of sand, and used hand sanitiser to clean myself up.

Jesus. I couldn't believe what had just happened. It must have been all the stress, sleep deprivation and highly processed foods I was consuming. My bowel had broken down.

I went to work commando that day, feeling shaken. What was this job doing to my body? I'd always been fit and healthy, so for me to lose such a basic bodily function was terrifying.

I wrote about the shit-show on Facebook. I knew I was over-sharing but I didn't care. I was really suffering and suddenly I couldn't do it alone. I was craving social interaction and some compassion. My post garnered a lot of comments: 'This is <bullshit / outrageous / terrible / ridiculous / insane / unfair / unsafe / shite>'. 'You should call in sick.' 'Your roster is illegal.' 'You need to leave your job.'

Reading the comments helped a little bit. At least they validated my experience, and that the horrors of this job were not just my perception. But in other ways the comments left me feeling even more helpless. There was no way I could quit now. Not after everything I'd already invested, and everything I'd sacrificed.

One friend put me in touch with a surgeon who was on a committee with RACS. I gave her a ring and told her what had been happening. 'What you're going through is totally unacceptable,' she said. 'But unfortunately, we can't help you because you're not on the Program. I only have the capacity to do something for accredited registrars.' Ah, yes. Another reminder of my failure. I felt like such a cast-off. No one cared about unaccredited registrars. We weren't good enough to be trained into specialists, and we didn't have any sort of representation.

My Facebook post must have got back to Dr Sansevieria because she rang me a few days later. I'd forgotten how small the medical community was.

'Oh, it's been absolutely awful,' I said, not holding back. 'This roster is too much.'

'I'll talk to Dr Nepenthes to discuss it,' she said. 'We've got to look after you. You're damn good, you're damn good.'

'Thank you,' I said, relieved.

'I don't want you to burn out,' she said.

Burnout. I didn't like that word. It had negative connotations, as though it was the person burning out who had the problem. I didn't want to be that person. I didn't want to be seen as 'acopic' – a word we use in Medicine to talk about people who aren't coping. But was I burning out? I was definitely exhausted, there was no doubt about that. I also felt distant and disconnected from the job I used to love. I thought about how I'd wanted to hurt my hand. Never in the past had I imagined ways to escape work. I'd lost the confidence I once had, too. I always knew I was good at my job, but I wasn't getting much encouragement this term. In a profession rife with nepotism, I'd made it to this stage without having any family members or friends in the medical profession. For this I was proud, but was it also going to be my undoing? If I'd had some inside knowledge on how toxic surgery really was, I'm not sure that I would've walked down this ostensibly manicured garden path. All I'd ever wanted was to perform operations that would save people's lives, or improve their quality of living. Why couldn't I simply do my job and be treated decently while I was doing it? Why these hoops to jump through, arses to kiss, and barriers that were impossible to break down? For the first time in my life, I doubted my survival. My education and commitment had brought me this far, but I wasn't sure that I could carry myself further.

The next evening Dr Nepenthes was performing surgery on a very complex hand fracture. The patient had injured himself at work so Dr Nepenthes would be paid a handsome amount through the Workers Compensation scheme. The cynical part of me wondered whether he would've bothered to come to the hospital if it hadn't been covered by workers comp. The surgery piqued my interest. The bone was shattered into a number of pieces and would need a combination of a plate and a few different screws to hold all the fragments together. I wanted to see how Dr Nepenthes would tackle this case, just in case I was ever on my own for a fracture this difficult to fix.

'Oh no, no, you go home,' he said. 'We wouldn't want you to get too tired, now, would we?' The sarcasm was piercing.

'I'm not tired. I'd like to stay,' I said. 'I want to learn from this case.'

I had raised my voice about the rostering and the consequences were already clear. My career was being ground to a fine crumble. I thought of Hajime battling the chemo. He'd always been my biggest career cheerleader. If he knew how much I was suffering now, he would be heartbroken.

When I got home that night I checked my mailbox. I had a late notice for my electricity and phone bills. It bothered me because I'd always been so organised and paid every bill on time. It was unlike me to be forgetful about anything.

The next day, I was working with an anaesthetist who wasn't keen on operating on a patient with a contagious bug called MRSA – the golden staph. The patient was on the medical ward, and had a large skin cancer on her chest that needed removal. 'The surgery won't take long,' I promised the anaesthetist. 'We can do it under a local anaesthetic with a bit of sedation.'

'But it's going to take such a long time to clean the theatre afterwards,' she said.

'This poor lady has already been cancelled a few times,' I said, finding myself slowly getting angry at the prospect of having to cancel her again.

I was sick of apologising to patients all the time; of waiting all day to get an operation done, only for the operating theatre to run out of time. The disheartening thing was that when patients did get deferred, I couldn't even guarantee their procedure would happen the next day, or the next.

I could feel hot tears rolling down my cheeks. I hated the fact that I was crying at work but I couldn't hold in my frustration.

'I'm just so fed up of cancelling all these patients,' I said to the scrub nurse next to me. She looked at me with sadness.

'The anaesthetist has no reason to cancel this lady,' I continued. 'She just can't be bothered with all the contact precautions like gowning up because the patient has MRSA. It's unfair.'

The anaesthetist looked over and saw me crying. 'Oh, so you're going to cry every time things don't go your way?' she huffed.

On Good Friday I had some surgeries to do. Hand surgeries, as usual. The nurse in charge was a young woman called Neveah, who was fairly new to her managerial role. She was unable to locate the first patient and called me in a tizzy. 'You didn't tell the patient where to go!' she yelled down the phone. 'It's *your* responsibility!'

I had told the patient exactly where to go for his admission but I didn't think arguing over the phone would be helpful, so I told her I'd sort it out and ended the conversation. It turned out the patient *had* gone to the right place, but the receptionist was unsure of where he should wait given that it was a public holiday and the pre-op area was closed.

All it took was a simple phone call to the patient to track him down: he was waiting in the foyer of the hospital. He informed me that Neveah had been quite unprofessional, ranting about how 'Plastics aren't doing their job.' I offered him an apology, but he took my side, remembering our conversation the night before in which I had given him clear instructions.

Soon we were underway for his surgery. When I walked up to the operating theatre I saw Neveah, who had forgotten about her earlier outrage and greeted me with an enthusiastic 'Hello!' I was in two minds about whether to say anything, but by this point in my term I was sick of how people were treating me, so I calmly said to Neveah, 'I don't appreciate how I was spoken to on the phone.' Her facial expression changed as soon as she remembered and she mumbled a quick 'Sorry.' I told her it was okay and tried to be understanding: she'd only been in this role a handful of times, and running the emergency theatre list was stressful. But at the same time, I didn't want her to talk to other registrars like that.

Easter Sunday was April Fool's Day. I'd been on call all week and it was a blistering hot day. Some friends were hanging out on Shelly Beach. I was stuck at the hospital, but I said I would try my best to join them, even if it was just for a quick 'hi'. That afternoon, I managed to get out of the hospital. I started driving towards the Northern Beaches. I hadn't been to Shelly Beach before, so I pulled over when I was nearly there to look at Google Maps, only to find my phone dead. I had charged it – surely it couldn't be depleted already. I turned it on and off in desperation. *Oh no. It can't die on me like this, not now. How am I supposed to receive hospital calls?* I definitely had to find my friends now – to borrow one of their phones.

I got to the beach the old-school way – I stopped someone on the footpath for directions. Eventually I made it, but I wasn't sure whether my friends would still be there. I anxiously scanned the beach like a metal detector for a few minutes, and finally saw them. *Bleep. Thank you, Jesus.* I ran over to them and asked for a phone immediately, then I called the hospital and requested the switchboard operator put me through to Amos.

'Amos, my phone's broken,' I said. 'Can I ask you to cover my calls for me until the morning?'

'I'm busy. You have to sort your own problems out,' he said.

Right. I'd been on call since Monday morning – seven straight days and nights – and he wouldn't even take a few calls through one night. No shops were open. There was nowhere I could go to buy myself a cheap replacement phone and a SIM card. What was I supposed to do?

'Can I come in a bit late on Tuesday so I can get my phone fixed?' I asked.

'Take time off when you're not working,' he said.

I rang the switchboard back and asked to be put through to the ENT registrar, Simon. I asked if he could cover my calls.

'I haven't done hand surgery before so I'm not comfortable taking your calls,' he said. *How do you think I feel about covering ENT?* Simon then remembered that he had a spare phone I could use. We decided to meet outside my apartment. As I thanked my friends and ran off, I tripped over a rock and scraped my foot – there was lots of blood and a piece of skin flapping up and down. It was as though it was clapping for me. *Well done, Yumiko, well done.* I was always running from one place to another, no time to stop. I was getting annoyed with myself for being so accident-prone.

Simon and I arrived at my apartment at the same time. I changed the SIM cards over and my heart sank as I saw how many calls I'd missed in the one hour since my phone had decided to die. The first thing I needed to do, though, was sort out my foot. I had some antiseptic, so I cleaned the wound with that and removed as much sand as I could see. As any good plastic surgery registrar does, I had a variety of sutures in my backpack and some local anaesthetic. Unfortunately I had no needles with which to administer the anaesthetic, so I sutured myself without it. I have a high pain tolerance, so it didn't hurt too much.

When I next looked at the phone I saw that Dr Demir had messaged me. He'd been called about a patient with a swollen parotid gland but he didn't trust the assessment of the ED doctor, so he asked if I would review the man as well. I wasn't sure what my assessment would add to this case, given my total lack of experience in ENT, but I drove to the hospital to admit the patient.

34

Emotional female

2018, Sydney

After the Easter weekend, Neveah found me in the operating theatre. She held up a large golden box of Ferrero Rocher chocolates. 'I'm so sorry for shouting at you,' she said. 'I kept thinking about it on the weekend. You've only ever been nice to me so I feel really bad.' That made *me* feel bad for making *her* feel bad! Of course I was upset about how she'd spoken to me, but I felt a little guilty that it had consumed her thoughts over the long weekend. The chocolates were unnecessary, but it was a lovely thing for Neveah to do. I thanked her and added them to my emergency snack supply in the registrars' office. After two months of dealing with constant unpleasantries, it seemed almost miraculous that at least one person had acknowledged their behaviour and wanted to make amends.

The following week, I took a day off to see my GP, Dr Perera. Having lost Akuto-san to cervical cancer I was diligent about getting my Pap smears, but other than that I hadn't needed to see her for much over the past few years. This was certainly the first time I'd visited her in such a distressed, emotional state. I told Dr Perera about my bowel accident on the way to work and how run down I felt. She'd known me for a few years, and she had never seen me like this before. She wrote a letter for me to take to the hospital, strongly recommending that they review my rostering.

Back at my apartment I scanned the letter and emailed it to the JMO manager and Dr Sansevieria. I also decided on my day off that I would draw up three alternative roster solutions. When I showed them to Dr Sansevieria, she thought they were all reasonable and said they would be discussed at the next consultant meeting. She didn't mention Dr Perera's letter.

The general surgeons, horrified by my roster, had got involved by this stage, too. The Head of Surgery was a general surgery professor, who reassured me that he would ensure the Plastic Surgery department changed the roster to make it fairer. I was partly relieved, partly disheartened, because I was pretty sure by now that my dream of becoming a surgeon was slipping away from me. With the rostering issue escalated, there was just no way I would have the support I needed for my application for the Program. I started to think, *should I keep going?* Even if I did get on to the training program, did I even still want it? This was unnavigated territory for me. Before now, I hadn't even fathomed a life without surgery. The idea filled me with trepidation.

I was back on call the next day and driving home in peak-hour traffic. I normally went home a bit later, so I hadn't realised how terrible traffic was at that time of day. I had been on the road for nearly two hours – the cars were barely moving.

I had two hand surgeries to do, but the anaesthetist had informed me that it was very unlikely I'd get them done that day – 'Definitely not before nine,' he'd said. The orthopods had booked some cases before mine. Knowing what things were like by now, it seemed inevitable I'd get cancelled and deferred until tomorrow.

I was one street away from my apartment when my phone rang.

'Hello, Yumiko speaking.'

'Oh Yumiko, it's theatres. The orthopaedic surgeon wants to do his cases tomorrow so you can do your case next.'

'What? I was told that I wouldn't be operating until at least nine pm, if at all.'

I couldn't believe those orthopods. They'd bumped my cases to the end of the list because theirs was more 'urgent'. But now that it was after five o'clock they'd decided that it wasn't urgent after all because they wanted to go home.

I did a U-turn and drove another two hours back in heavy traffic. As I finished operating on the first patient, who had a tendon injury, the dreaded moment came. I would not get to do my other case. I was extra-frustrated because the second surgery was a nerve repair, which would not have taken me long. The gastroenterologist had called theatre to book an urgent gastroscopy that would have to be done after my current case. So, as per usual, my second surgery got cancelled for me to do the next day. Time for me to issue another apology.

I was exhausted from all the driving, so I immediately fell asleep that night. A few hours later, my phone rang. An Emergency registrar was calling to book an appointment for a wound review. I looked at my clock. Three am.

'It's three in the morning,' I said. 'I'm on call for emergencies. This is not an emergency.'

'We need your approval before we can book patients into your clinic,' he said.

'Yes, but you don't need to call at three a.m. for that,' I replied.

'It's our protocol.'

'And you couldn't wait to contact me in the morning?' I asked, getting wound up as this conversation unrolled.

'It's not a big deal – you say "yes", then you go back to sleep,' he said.

'It *is* a big deal. Surgical registrars do twenty-four-hour on-call shifts. When *you* finish work, you get to go home and sleep. In a few hours I have to go back and work a full day. When we get calls in the middle of the night it fucks us up the next day.'

'Calm down, you're being an emotional female,' he said.

'Excuse me?' I was furious. 'Don't call for non-urgent matters at this time again.'

I hung up, and my heart was beating in my ears. How dare he call me emotional! If Amos had said the same thing, would he have called *him* emotional?

I felt even worse about the phone call later that week because the patient didn't turn up for his appointment. After opening up the file, it turned out that he had actually sustained a burn, which the ED registrar had failed to mention. Due to our lack of nursing staff to do burns dressings, the hospital did not accept burns referrals. These were normally sent to another hospital that had a well-established burns unit. I was unimpressed. That patient should never have been referred to me in the first place, but he was, I was woken up at 3 am for it, and now he hadn't shown up to his appointment.

Being miserably tired had become my normal state of being. Not even my first coffee for the day could perk me up, but I tried to see each morning as an opportunity to reset how I felt. After the ward round, I would check up on Mr Pilea, the elderly patient with the finger infection. His recovery was slow but the finger was definitely getting better. Before walking in I always made sure I had a bright smile on my face.

'Good morning, Mr Pilea,' I greeted him.

'Good morning, Yumiko. How are you?' he asked. It was such a rare thing for me to get asked how I was, but Mr Pilea never failed to enquire.

'I'm fine, thank you,' I replied. 'Today I have some positive news. The results from yesterday show that your infection is getting better. The white blood cells, which go up during an infection, are in the normal range now.'

'Oh, that's great,' he said. 'My finger looks much better too.'

'It really does. I don't think you'll need daily dressings for much longer.'

'Can I ask you a question?' he asked.

'Of course,' I replied.

'You've seen me every day for several weeks, even on weekends. Doesn't this affect your family life?' he asked. I was surprised. I was expecting a clinical question about his finger.

'Yes, but it's okay. I love my job,' I said.

'You've been my guardian angel,' he said.

The truth was, Mr Pilea was mine. His kindness made my heart swell with gratitude. No matter how horrible I felt in those weeks, I looked forward to seeing Mr Pilea in the mornings. He was always so pleasant, and made me feel good about my job, that I was actually doing something that made a difference. My daily interaction with him was the only constant in my life, and I was grateful. If it weren't for him, the previous weeks would have been much harder to tolerate.

Yoshiko sent me a picture of a chest X-ray. Hajime was getting admitted to hospital with a huge amount of fluid around his right lung. I was surprised he could even breathe. The X-ray was quite dramatic, and looking at it made me feel guilty that I wasn't with my parents. I was tempted to quit the hospital right now and fly over there, but of course quitting would have massive repercussions. I would never have a job in Plastic Surgery in Sydney. It was a small community, and once surgeons find out that you've broken a contract, you are deemed undependable. Nina hadn't actually broken her contract when she'd gone back to England and I recalled the bullying she was subjected to. But at this stage, honestly, I didn't care. More and more I was becoming convinced that after all these years, all this training, perhaps I wasn't going to succeed after this disaster of a term. It was so messed up.

I called Maxence, whom I had assisted last year. He was one of the few plastic surgeons I knew who didn't work in the public hospital system. I needed to talk to someone who was distanced from it.

'Maxence,' my voice trembled on the phone, 'I don't know how much longer I can do this. This term is just awful.'

'Oh Yumes, I know,' he said. 'You just need to think about what you want in the long run.' It was easy for him to say.

Maxence was now a successful surgeon with a doting wife at home.

'I don't know if I want this anymore,' I said. 'I think I've hit my limit.'

'We've all had those horror terms,' he said. 'Some of my registrar years were so bad that I've completely blacked them out from my memory.'

'I just can't imagine how I can physically see out this term,' I said.

'Look, if you want to have kids in the future, it's really hard,' he said. 'Maybe it's not a bad thing to leave. You do what's right for you.'

My career had always come first, so kids were the last thing on my mind. I'd put the whole idea in the 'too hard' basket after seeing Bernadette and others struggling with motherhood and Medicine. It was just easier to repeat 'knife before life' ad nauseam to drown out any thoughts of a normal, happy, life – whatever that might be. Besides, I had one slight prerequisite missing: I had no one to have children with.

First thing in the morning on Friday the first of June I checked my emails to see if Amos had sent a roster for the remainder of term. He had. Amos and Simon were taking annual leave. I would be working nineteen consecutive days in June, and twenty-one straight days in July.

When I arrived at work I started the ward round with Kevin and Thea, just like any other day. I had admitted a few patients overnight who were new to the ward – one had a hand injury, another a jaw infection and he was already on the way to the operating theatre. The man with the hand injury looked at Kevin.

'What's happening?' he asked. 'Do you think I need an operation?'

'Yumiko is the registrar,' said Kevin, pointing at me. 'She makes the plans.'

'Oh,' said the patient, turning to look at me.

'Yes, you do need surgery. Your X-ray showed a broken bone which will need some wires, and you have an open wound that we need to clean and close,' I explained.

After the ward round, I rang Dr Nepenthes, who was on call. I updated him on the patients and asked if he would like to see the CT scan of the patient with the jaw infection.

'No, you explained it well enough,' he said. 'You know what you need to do?'

'Yes. I'll approach it from the buccal side of the mandible,' I explained, picturing the procedural steps in my head. 'I'll go down the sub-periosteal plane until I reach the infection along the inferior edge.'

'Good.'

A few years ago, this sort of operation would have intimidated me. Now, I felt fine about doing it, but it held no excitement. I felt a little nostalgic about my early registrar years. There was a time when everything was new, including a case like this. It was thrilling. Now, what should have felt exciting didn't feel like anything.

I walked into the anaesthetic bay to greet the patient.

'I'm nearly ready to operate on you,' I said. 'We'll wheel you inside in a moment.'

'Oh,' he said. 'Are *you* doing the operation?'

'Yes,' I said. 'Do you remember me from before?' I thought perhaps this man had been on such strong painkillers that he had forgotten my face. I had spent time obtaining his informed consent for the surgery, as well as seen him on my ward round.

'Yeah, I do remember you,' he said. 'I thought you were a nurse.'

Why was it so inconceivable that a woman could possibly be their surgeon? I was already baseline irritated from the sleep deprivation, and that comment only made me feel worse. I went to the storeroom to look for equipment and found the scout nurse there, gathering instruments.

'You look terrible,' she said. 'Are you okay?' That was the first time anyone had asked me all term whether I was okay. I burst into tears.

'No . . . no, I'm not,' I said, the tears dropping onto my pale blue top, making darker blue splotches on it. 'I've been working for twenty-four days in a row, and I don't think I can keep going.'

'I'm so sorry,' she said. That's all anyone could really say. That they were sorry for me. As much as I appreciated the sympathy, sorry couldn't fix anything.

I wiped my tears, washed my face, and walked back into the operating theatre. I couldn't even force a smile. I felt like a robot doing surgery. Bite block. Blade. Periosteal elevator. The words came out of my mouth, then my hands did the talking. After the operation, I went to find Dr Sansevieria who was operating in the adjacent theatre.

'I'm utterly exhausted,' I told her. 'Please. Will you let me go home early today?'

'Just hang on,' she said.

I felt like I'd been hanging on for four months. I didn't think I could hang on any longer. I was physically depleted and spiritually broken. I rang the JMO manager.

'Hello, is that rostering?'

'Yes, how can I help you?'

'Hello, it's Yumiko. I'm calling to ask what the minimum notice is to resign.'

I was done. I'd submitted my resignation by email. On the way home in my car I could barely stay awake, but I thought I was going to make it back until . . . Crunch. The traffic lights turned green and I'd reversed into the car behind me. For a split second I was confused. I looked down at my idiot left hand, which was clinging tightly to the gear stick. *What the fuck did you do?* I just stared at R, N and D. Reverse, Neutral, Drive. How on earth had I moved gear to Reverse? It was as if my brain was not connected to my hand. I opened my bag on the passenger seat and grabbed my driver's licence out of my wallet. I wanted to drill a large pothole into the asphalt and bury myself in it. I got out of the car to apologise to the driver behind me and exchange details.

When I got home, I ran the shower. I sat on the tiles and let the water stream over my head. I let out a guttural scream and cried, my tears as one with the water. I could not move. I don't know how long I sat underneath that shower. It might have been an hour. I didn't know how to feel. I was angry. Relieved. Regretful. Happy. Devastated. I was all of those, and none of those at the same time. I was numb.

One of the first things I thought was, *I can't wait to go to the gym*. Then I went through my mental list of everything I wanted to do that had been put on hold because of my pursuit of the Program. I wanted to see my family, do more yoga, go running. I planned on taking a week to rest, and then I'd throw myself back into activities. I expected this was just a small bump in the road.

Suddenly all was quiet. I could finally lie down. Not get interrupted by phone calls. I could switch my phone to silent mode. My pager was no longer attached to my waist band. My room was so still I could only hear the hum of my refrigerator and the occasional *ding* of the elevators going up and down my apartment building.

RING. My phone. I rolled over and reached for it. But no one was calling. It was on silent, yet I could still hear its ringtone bashing at my eardrums. I was in a mental tundra. Once, I'd felt every emotion like they were colours in the Pantone catalogue. Not now. I was emotionally destitute and trapped in a bleak monochrome darkness. My brain was disabled. Every movement felt heavy. I lay in the anatomical position, on my back, palms facing up, empty eyes staring at the ceiling, beckoning an answer. Why did this happen?

35

Aparigraha

2018, Sydney to Bali

Dr Sansevieria rang about my resignation that same evening.

'Can't you just see out this term? It's only another couple of months,' she said.

'No, I don't think I can,' I said.

'It's a shame,' she said. 'You're good at what you do. You have good hands. But if you can't handle the hours, I guess this isn't for you.'

I went to sleep. You'd think that being so exhausted I'd have had the best sleep of my life. But no. When I woke up it was still dark. I thought that maybe it was 5 am. I looked over at my clock. Midnight. When I woke up again, it was 1 am. I woke up every hour like clockwork.

*

The first people I told about my situation were my sisters. Both Eriko and Mariko were shocked, but they understood. Eriko set up a three-way video call and we talked for an hour. I asked both of them to promise not to tell our parents. I wasn't ready. I could barely face even the *idea* of telling them, in fact. I didn't want to disappoint them after everything they'd done to put me through medical school. All the financial support, as well as the cheerleading. I didn't want to worry them. Hajime was still going through chemotherapy. There was just no way I could put this sort of stress on to them.

I was supposed to see out four more weeks, but the following Monday I realised that I couldn't possibly make myself go to the hospital. Even though I was so tired, I had barely slept the past three nights. And I was filled with a dread that even now is hard to describe. I went to see Dr Perera and burst into tears.

'I can't do this,' I sobbed, my shoulders shaking violently. 'I handed in my notice on Friday but I can't do the four weeks.'

Dr Perera was concerned about my mental health and decided to refer me to a psychiatrist. I reluctantly accepted the referral. I didn't think I had a mental health issue. However, I was desperate to feel better. I wanted something that would help me sleep and help me regain my energy.

At the appointment I was greeted by Dr Pal, a lady with a short bob and thick-rimmed glasses. She motioned to me to sit down, and just let me talk. My words poured out in an incoherent heap. I didn't even know where to begin, but eventually it all emerged – my harrowing experience at the hospital. I was an ugly crier. My face was red and swollen. I helped myself to her tissue box, dabbed my face and blew my nose.

After finishing my story, Dr Pal looked at me empathetically. 'Yumiko, what an awful thing you've been through. I used to work at the Medical Board and I thought these hours were ancient history.'

She then delivered me my diagnosis: depression.

'What? Oh no, *no no no no no no no no*. I can't have depression. No way. I'm a happy person. I'm just tired right now,' I said.

Dr Pal went through the diagnostic criteria with me and of course she was right – it appeared I was quite severely depressed. I hadn't paid any attention to my symptoms because I was so pummelled by work. The only thing that had alerted me to something being seriously wrong was when I'd lost faecal continence. I ignored other things, such as losing interest in activities I used to enjoy, because I couldn't prioritise them. Who cares if I hadn't gone to yoga in a long time when I was only just able to manage the horrendous hours at the hospital?

'I am going to start you on a mild antidepressant called Valdoxan. It works on the melatonin receptors so it should also help you with your sleep, which I know is your biggest concern right now.'

It was one thing to accept that I was suffering depression, quite another to think about medication. I didn't even take paracetamol unless I really had to. Yet if Valdoxan was going to help me sleep, in the end I decided I was willing to take it. I was desperate for even just one good night's rest.

The Valdoxan didn't work. Over the winter months we tried various antidepressants and sleep medications. I was having ups and downs but, overall, I wasn't really getting better, which frightened me. What's wrong with my body? Why isn't it normal?

I'm sure it being winter didn't help. I was grasping at hypotheses as to why I wasn't right. I needed my sisters more than I ever had in the past. I knew that if they were in Sydney, I wouldn't allow them to see me like this. They wouldn't allow it either. We don't throw pity parties; we never have. They'd pick me up and get me out of the house to do fun activities. That's what I needed. I FaceTimed them to organise them to come over for my birthday in August, which, conveniently, was coming up.

I was also panicking about my future. What was I going to do? I'd studied for six years, and worked for nearly eight. I had expected to be better by now, and I needed to get on with my life; also, I felt more clearly than I had in June that I couldn't just throw away a surgical career. There was no way I was going to get a job in plastic surgery so I thought hard about what my other options were. My favourite term was the Children's Hospital. The care of kids with burns was shared between Plastic Surgery and Paediatric Surgery, so it made sense that I try to get back to Burns via the paediatric surgery stream. I called Uncle Phil to talk to him about what had happened, without going too much into the mental health side of things. I wasn't ready to talk about that yet. It was easier to say I 'burned out'. I discussed restarting my career in paediatric surgery, given how much I'd loved working with him at the Children's Hospital. He was supportive of this plan and agreed to be a referee. 'Yep, happy to help,' he said. Happy to help. I paused on his words, and let them echo in my head. Happy to help. Someone was happy to help me.

I applied for a few jobs in paediatric surgery – also because I didn't know what to do with myself when I wasn't working. And then I ordered a textbook online – *Jones' Clinical Paediatric*

Surgery: Diagnosis and Management. I was knowledgeable in paediatric burns management, but I knew there were other areas in paediatric surgery that I would need to brush up on. If I was giving myself another chance to succeed in surgery, I was going to get back into it, full guns ablazing.

I spoke to my sisters about my new plans. Apart from Uncle Phil, I didn't talk to anyone else, though. I didn't know who was a good or bad guy anymore, so it was safer to put everyone in the 'bad guy' category to protect myself. Mariko told me to just 'chill'. But I didn't know how. What was I supposed to do? But I decided that she was probably right. If I was going to go back to work I'd need to restore my energy. So I did some online research to help me create a contingency plan on how to 'chill'. I took my carefully curated list with me to the shops to gather some goods to execute this plan. Winter was a good time to take a bath, I thought. What do people who are 'chill' put in their baths? Perhaps some lavender essential oil. I also ticked off chamomile tea and scented candles, and went home armed with my armamentarium of 'chill'.

The bath tub was dusty, me never having used it in all the years of living in my apartment. Could I really be bothered to clean it? I was already regretting carrying through Mariko's advice. Chilling was too cumbersome. I swished some water around to give the tub a quick rinse, and then ran the bath. This better be worth it. I started to feel agitated as the water level slowly climbed. This was taking too long. What was I supposed to do while the tub was filling? I couldn't just sit there. I went online to track my paediatric surgery textbook to see when it would be arriving, and then checked my emails. A message from Dr Bruno about our article. Urgh. I couldn't deal with that. My reflexes slammed my laptop shut. I put the kettle on. I suppose I should try out this chamomile tea, I thought. While the kettle was boiling, I unpacked the lavender oil and took a sniff. It just reminded me of air fresheners, like they use in toilets. When I finally got into the bath it was too hot. I lasted all of thirty seconds before hopping out and taking a shower. I unplugged the bath and watched the water swirl clockwise down the hole, and thought about how my own world had spun off its axis.

The medical community being small, word had spread that I had resigned. I received a text message from Dr Whiteley asking how I was doing. I was honest with her and told her that I was suffering from depression.

'Well, of course you are,' she said. 'All that exercise you used to do. You've lost all your endorphins.'

'That's true,' I said, realising that that must have had some effect on my brain chemistry. It was an easy theory to understand, if only it were that simple. It was also less confronting than talking about the punishing conditions that had led me to where I was. Besides, she knew Dr Sansevieria, so I was guarded. Not that it mattered anymore. I could've gone full-on savage about the hospital, and if it had been relayed back to the hospital I didn't care.

She asked if I wanted to come to assist her in the private hospital again. I wasn't sure. That felt like a backward step. I didn't want to go back to the doldrums of 2016. I also remained cautious about other people, especially surgeons. I hadn't decided yet who I could trust again but I strongly felt that the way to get my career back on track was to find a full-time job in a public hospital. In the end I avoided the issue by telling Dr Whiteley I had other job interviews.

'Normal people with depression don't go to job interviews,' she said. 'Only you.'

I didn't know how to take that. I hoped she meant it as a compliment on my resilience, but I felt she may have also been questioning my validity. Did she think I was faking it?

I did well in my interviews and I was offered a paediatric surgery job. However, I ended up declining it because, when it came to the crunch, it was clear I wasn't ready to work again. I knew I wouldn't be able to cope with the sound of pagers beeping and phones ringing. I still could barely respond to my own phone. My heart would start beating nervously every time I saw 'No Caller ID', because it reminded me of the hospital switchboard. And I continued to hear the phone ringing when it wasn't. I was taunted by post-traumatic symptoms almost every day. Dr Perera also practically forbade my return, telling me that realistically she couldn't see me back to any hospital environment for at least a year.

A year? I was in disbelief. It was as though I wasn't really in my body. Was any of this real? Panicking again about my future, I called Uncle Phil to ask his advice: do I try to get back into plastic surgery again? I thought about all the years, the blood, sweat, and tears I'd spent working towards this dream.

'To tell you the truth,' he began, 'I don't think you'll get another job in Sydney. If you really want to do plastic surgery, you might have to go to Brisbane or Melbourne.'

As I'd feared. I'd black-listed myself in Sydney.

'If I can give you some advice,' he continued. 'You're a very emotional person . . .'

'Yes . . .'

'You might want to tone that down around surgeons,' he said. 'I'm sure that that's what makes you a good human, and a good doctor to your patients. But surgeons will see that you're emotional and consider it a weakness.'

'I don't know what to do,' I said, feeling a lump rising in my throat.

'You need to get better first,' he said. 'Get better first and then we can talk about your next career move. Okay, kiddo?'

'Okay.'

There were days when I couldn't get out of bed, except to go to the toilet. I felt flat, drained, like a car that had had its lights on all night. I wished someone could just jump-start me. I was thirty years old. I had been to a number of thirtieth birthday parties in the past year, celebrating friends who had achieved so much. One was a Rhodes scholar. Many had already finished their training programs and were fully fledged GPs. I realised that's how I had been measuring success: whether or not you had qualified in your chosen field. To me, I was a failure. I had never got on to the Program.

For my own thirtieth, I'd had a small dinner, and I didn't want any speeches because I didn't feel as though I'd accomplished anything. I thought I would have been more by thirty. More this. More that. Just more. I thought I'd be well on my way to becoming a surgeon. For nearly half my life, I'd been in Medicine. And yet what had it all led to? Nothing. I felt I was nothing.

Some days I browsed the internet, living vicariously through people holidaying in Bali. As it was winter in Sydney, I daydreamed about sipping from a fresh coconut on a beach. I needed to fix myself, so, I thought, what would make me feel better? A lot of yoga, perhaps. I still remembered the very first yoga class I'd attended when I was an intern and Martha had taken me to the bikram yoga studio. That was nearly ten years ago, I realised. My body had felt so energised then. I wanted that feeling back.

Never one to do things by halves, I decided that throwing myself into an intensive yoga-teacher course might give me what I needed. I needed to find the Yin to my Cristina Yang. I started researching various programs in and around Bali. I had worked hard and saved my wages since I was an intern, but still, I was concerned that if I went overseas I had no job to return to. Was I being frivolous? Fuck it. I'd been putting patients first. It was about time I did something for myself. I needed to give myself permission to be selfish. I also desperately wanted to see my sisters.

I found a yoga course in Nusa Lembongan, a small island off the east coast of Bali, and a week before I left, Eriko and Mariko flew over from Tokyo to spend some time with me in Sydney. We had a great week and I began to feel a bit more myself again. We pampered ourselves with pedicures and facials for some 'chill'. We played upbeat songs and danced in my living room with face masks on. We went to see a musical. We went out for brunches and dinners. We cycled in parks, and along the water. We did yoga and coastal walks. What a stunning city I lived in. It was like rediscovering Sydney. There was so much to do, and so much nature to appreciate. I was having fun and my sisters made me forget I was depressed. I was starting to see that life could be enjoyable. The time felt far too short when I had to say goodbye to them.

I was apprehensive about going to Lembongan. What were the other yogis going to be like? Would they be like the yogis on Instagram? Would they be wearing expensive activewear and be able to do handstands and other fancy poses that I couldn't do? Was I audacious for thinking I was good enough to become a teacher?

I caught a boat to the island from Sanur on the mainland. The sea was choppy and this tiny speedboat bopped over the giant waves like a fragile, dancing marionette. After a while, I saw brightly coloured beach houses and the comforting yellow of shore. When I jumped off the boat I felt the tepid water around my legs. Aquamarine and clear. A perfect painting. My legs were unsteady as my toes tried to dig into the wet sand. *I made it.*

Being close to Indonesia, there were, predictably, a few Australians on the island. The rest of the group had travelled afar. From the United States there was a soon-to-be-married couple, Alice and Patrick; a Californian girl, Heather; and Emily. Luisa was there from Brazil. From Europe were Birta 'Bee' from Iceland, Jessica from Germany and Kati from Austria. Yasmin and Chiara were medical students from Italy, and Julienne was an intensive care doctor who lived in Guam. I decided not to tell anyone that I was a doctor. I wanted nothing to do with Medicine. I was there to do lots of yoga. No one needed to know about my life in Sydney.

On the first day of this month-long course, we gathered in the yoga studio, called a shala. It was a brightly lit space with the sun streaming through large windows, and surrounded by birds of paradise and banana trees. We started with an ashtanga yoga class led by our main teacher Gwen, a tall Frenchwoman with long brown hair. She had a mandala tattooed in one elbow crease and marine-themed tattoos scattered on the rest of her arms. Her class was difficult. I knew that yoga was about focusing on oneself, but I couldn't help but look around. I was intimidated by Luisa, who had a strong physique and effort-lessly moved between the advanced poses. She looked like she had been doing ashtanga for a very long time. I hadn't done this style of yoga before so I struggled. Being naturally flexible, I normally found yoga easy, but I was unexpectedly challenged. There were poses that made my joints move into places they'd never been before. The competitive side of me was frustrated.

Later that morning we had our first philosophy class. Our teacher was Lisa, a bubbly Canadian woman with wild blonde hair, a nose ring, and tattooed sleeves on her arms. Yoga philosophy had its roots in Hinduism, but the teachings were universal – not harming others, for example. It reminded me of medical ethics, one of the pillars being non-maleficence: first, do no harm. Lisa introduced us to the *yamas* and *niyamas*, which are principles by which to live. The *yamas* are restraints, the *niyamas* observances. Our homework was to think of some *yamas* and *niyamas* that applied to us in our lives, as well as on the yoga mat.

I chose *aparigraha* as one of the *yamas* to study. *Aparigraha* means disidentification, or detachment from external factors and material possessions. It forced me to think about what formed my identity. I realised that I had spent so much of the past decade thinking of myself only as a surgeon-to-be. And so, of course, when I quit my job I lost my sense of self. *Who am I when I'm not being a surgeon? What will my life be without surgery?* It was difficult for me to separate myself from my vocation. I'd always been Yumiko the plastic surgery registrar. I answered to 'Plastics' for the past few years. Now what was I? I was having an identity crisis.

I read about the *niyamas*, and dwelled on *isvara pranidhana*, which means surrender to the universe. Did all of this happen for a reason? Maybe it was time to relinquish control and see where life would take me. This was something I'd never done before. I'd always had a path. But now that I was off it, and so far from the recent stress and mayhem, I didn't know if, when or how I would get back onto it. I had no handbook to follow. Did I even *want* to get back onto it, or was I possibly ready to let it all go?

Whenever I wondered that, the same fears came surging back at me: *it's not like I can do anything else. I don't have any other qualifications. I'm not naturally gifted at anything.* What else *was* I going to do?

36

Snakes and ladders

2018, Nusa Lembongan

One day we had a group discussion about yoga philosophy. The other yogis seemed friendly enough but I closed off. I felt a great need to protect myself. The past few months had made me recoil from others. I had deleted all of my social media accounts. I didn't want to see other people's highlight reels and successes. I was ashamed of myself and I had nothing to share with the world. I wanted to pour the events of the past year into a glass bottle and throw it out to sea.

Slowly, as we went around the class, my heart started pounding hard in my chest. Despite everything, I suddenly had an urge to share what had happened to me. They were all strangers. Perhaps that's what made it easier. Even if they did judge me, I wouldn't have to see them again after I left the island.

Initially, I spoke matter-of-factly about my job. The *niyama* of *tapas* was about discipline and dedication. That was easy enough to talk about. I then shared my reflections from the night before about identity, and that's when I lost control of my emotions. I started crying, which shocked me. I didn't think I was still feeling the grief of walking away from my career that strongly. I felt like I'd reopened a wound. The room became silent. Not even a flicker of a page or a click of a pen. There were a few tears on some of their faces. Suddenly I felt an incredible bond – I was in a safe space, surrounded by strangers who were transforming into new friends. To break the silence I decided to tell the group about the time I shat myself in the car. 'I was literally sitting in a pile of my own shit!' I exclaimed and laughed.

At morning tea time, the group sat around a large wooden table. I had a smoothie bowl inside a coconut shell. The dragon fruit created a vibrant fuchsia, and it was sprinkled with granola, almonds, cacao chips and banana. It was delicious and comforting. We ate in silence, until Jessica spoke up.

'Thank you for sharing your story,' she said. 'You are so brave.'

'Yes, thank you,' said Bee. 'I feel like it's changed the dynamic of the group.'

'I feel like the group is closer now,' said Kati. 'Can we give you a hug?'

One by one these lovely yogis from around the world stood up from their seats and embraced me. I'd forgotten how it felt to receive hugs, and I got sixteen one after the other. There was power in physical touch. I no longer felt like I was going through this course alone. I had made fast friends who were going to support me during this phase of my life. I knew these ladies would help me to trust other people again. I had to unlearn the fear that people had ulterior motives or malicious intent. It was hard to break down these beliefs, but the more time I spent with these women, the more it restored my faith in other humans.

That afternoon we had a session of restorative yoga with Gwen. Alice called it a 'guided nap', which was pretty accurate. I wasn't aware of this sort of yoga. When I started yoga, I liked the calming effect of it, of course, but what I really wanted to get out of it was a workout. I wanted to feel that I'd done something physically hard. The concept of relaxing had always been a bit foreign to me. As Mariko would say to me, 'Girl, you have no chill.'

We were set up in a reclined seated pose, held up by blocks and bolsters. We had blankets over us and an eye pillow. We were to sit in this pose for twenty minutes. Was this really yoga? I found it impossible to relax. My mind was racing with random thoughts. I tried to recall the opening chant of ashtanga yoga, which we had to memorise in Sanskrit. *Vande gurunam caranara vinde.* I thought about the smoothie bowl I wanted to order tomorrow. I wondered where Emily had bought her yoga mat. My legs were twitching. Being forced to sit still for twenty minutes was harder than I expected. It was not enjoyable at all. I wanted to take the eye pillow off my face and get up.

Every night was the same. I woke up every hour or two, and inevitably at 5 am I'd decide it wasn't worth trying to get back to sleep. One early morning I walked underneath the large leaves of the banana trees lining the path to the shala. At the front of the shala was a porch, and Luisa was the first one there. She sat fully captured by a book in her hands. I noticed she wore some beautiful gold rings on her fingers and a lovely chain around her neck with a moon and stars. Luisa was a jewellery designer in Brazil and had already been teaching yoga for a number of years.

'Can I ask you a question about the anatomy?' she asked, as I stepped out of my flip-flops and onto the porch.

'Yes, of course.' I sat down next to her. It was nice that I could offer Luisa something.

Just like that, we bonded every morning. I would ask her about yoga, and she would ask me about anatomy. It was a comfort to have her constantly there. I'd be up at 5 every morning, and I knew that Luisa would be sitting on the porch waiting. As the days went on I felt more comfortable opening up to her. I confided in her about my mental health, which she listened to without judgement. She introduced me to alternative therapies, like the ancient practice of Ayurveda, which encourages people to heal through dietary changes and meditation, among other holistic lifestyle choices. Even though Western medicine rejects such practices, a lot of people around the world seek alternative therapies and find benefit in them. I've always believed that we shouldn't 'yuk other people's yum'. Even if I didn't understand Ayurveda within the scientific paradigm I grew up with, Luisa's experience was valid. She helped me to be more open-minded about how people choose to heal themselves.

Afternoon classes were arduous. Because I wasn't sleeping well at night, I was exhausted after lunch each day and often fell asleep in class. There were some afternoons I was so tired that I retreated to my room and didn't come out for dinner. The women were very caring and understanding. Kati and Heather would save some dinner for me and bring it to my room whenever they noticed my absence. Some days were worse than others, but overall I felt I was healing. My mind was enriched by the philosophy classes, my body was getting stronger with every ashtanga session, and my spirits were lifting with every interaction I had with the women there. I was starting to laugh more, genuinely, deep from my belly. I was even starting to enjoy the restorative yoga sessions. Each time, I was able to relax a little bit longer. It wasn't easy for me, but slowly I let go and allowed my body to rest.

As the end of the course drew near, I felt nervous about going back to Sydney. While I had a structured program, it was easy for me to practise yoga every day. The food was catered, so I didn't need to worry about cooking. I felt supported by my new friends. What would happen when I returned? I wasn't sure whether I could keep up this healthy routine. I didn't want to leave this paradise. While I was in Nusa Lembongan it was easy for me to avoid thinking about my career conundrum. I wasn't exactly sure what my next move was going to be when I returned. I thought about the image of a ladder that we were shown at the beginning of medical school. Our career paths were clearly delineated on each rung. First, we were medical students, then interns, then residents. We would enter training programs as registrars in our chosen specialties, and after completion we would be consultants. I had fallen off my ladder and didn't know how to get back on. A small part of me still wanted to pursue surgery. It would be a waste not to. I had the knowledge and skills. I had come so far . . . but when would I be ready to throw myself back into the circus? Which surgical specialty should I re-enter? Should I stick to my new plan of paediatric surgery or try my luck in plastic surgery again?

If I persisted with plastics, should I go interstate, or even overseas? These were questions I still had.

Alice, Patrick and Heather were all in a similar position, having just walked away from their marketing and business careers. They were staying in the huts next to mine, so we spent a lot of time talking on our front porches. We were all at crossroads, contemplating what would happen next. We'd recognised that we needed a break from our lives and had come together on this small island to think about the big questions. It was comforting to know that there were others having a parallel experience, albeit in different fields. The common ground we shared was that we wanted to lead happier, more balanced lives. It felt very un-Japanese of me. So much of Japanese culture is about working hard, but I knew that I needed to be more self-compassionate. I needed to give myself permission to breathe. I needed to let go of my shame, but I didn't know if I could do that. The shame felt permanent.

On our final day in Lembongan, I hung out with Heather. She took a swig of her Bintang beer as she filled me in on her plans to visit Ubud next, in the central rainforests of Bali. I so wished I could join her for more yoga there. I couldn't believe I was having these thoughts. Just a month ago I'd arrived with no intentions of making any connections, and now I had made such wonderful friends I wanted to spend more time with them. Luisa gifted me a gold ring that she had designed. It was simple, elegant, beautiful, made of two intertwining lines. All of her jewellery designs were yoga-inspired. The two lines represented *ida* and *pingala*, which are the energy channels connected to our breathing. It was her reminder to me: 'Yumiko, don't forget to breathe,' she said. I was so touched by the gift. When I gave her a hug, I truly felt she was someone I had made a soul connection with. Throughout my few weeks at the retreat, Luisa had been such a calming influence. She was there every morning, reading quietly on the porch. Even when we didn't talk, we kept each other company while waiting for the morning class to start. I was going to miss her.

Later that afternoon we received our final results. I was worried that I would fail based on attendance because I had slept through many classes. When my name was called, it was such a triumph. Psychologically, it was a big deal to hold my yoga teacher certificate. It had only been a couple of months since quitting surgery. Giving up my career made me feel like a failure. That piece of paper told me I had succeeded in something else; that I was good enough.

Back in Sydney, I was able to keep up my new habits. I practised yoga every morning on my balcony. I made smoothie bowls at home that were just like the ones in Lembongan. I was so glad I had made the trip. I did something just for me, and it was changing my life for the better. I felt healthy, that my energy was returning. My bones didn't feel so heavy anymore. My footsteps felt lighter. My soul felt lighter. I still wasn't sleeping, but life was improving. I was excited to share my new skills with my sisters. I called Mariko on FaceTime and gave her my first yoga class. 'This is so cool!' she said. She was always so encouraging.

Later that week I decided I wanted to write about all of the things I'd learned in Lembongan. I had many new insights about yoga, and about lifestyle in general. The yogis on the course had inspired me to start eating more healthily. Most of them were vegan. I wasn't exactly sure if I'd be able to go completely vegan, but I decided to try. I kept in touch with Bee and Heather, who had both been vegan for a long time. They introduced me to nutritional yeast flakes, which were fortified with vitamin B12. 'Sprinkle them on everything! It's like cheese!' they said.

I had fancied starting a blog in my twenties, but I was never good with computers, or technology in general, so it hadn't eventuated. Besides, I was never going to be like one of those fabulous fashion bloggers with their photographer boyfriends and exotic location shoots. I did, however, like to write. I looked at several domains and hosting platforms and eventually set up a blog page. I wrote about my new plant-based diet and yoga. It was an escape from medical writing. I had been avoiding the article on breast cancer with Dr Bruno. I felt bad for ignoring him, but I just couldn't deal with anything remotely medical. A lot of the time I wanted to forget that I was a doctor.

So I did well for a few weeks, but I soon felt I was losing a grip on my new lifestyle. It started with the dishes. I couldn't be bothered to wash them, so I let them pile up in the sink. Clothes were strewn all over the floor like a multi-colour patchwork quilt. I couldn't see the carpet because there was stuff everywhere. I was getting swallowed in my squalor. I couldn't be bothered to cook. The smoothie bowls became tedious, so I resorted to eating muesli for every meal. Sometimes, if I was feeling adventurous, I'd go to the frozen food aisle of the supermarket and get myself some microwave meals.

Depression was a Dementor from Harry Potter sucking the life out of me. I was trudging through sand with my legs tied together. Yoga in Lembongan had been a momentary oasis in this desert of mine. Now I realised that it wasn't enough. Studying Eastern philosophy had helped me reframe my thinking, but it hadn't fixed my body. I was reminded that depression was an organic, neurochemical disease. Serotonin. Noradrenaline. What were those chemicals doing in my head? Clearly, they were still imbalanced. I needed to be patient with myself, as I would with any of my own patients. My brain had received a heavy hit, and a short course of yoga wasn't going to repair the damage overnight. But how long was it going to take?

My sense of healing diminished and I started to feel increasingly tired. The fatigue was familiar and there was nothing I could do to stop it. It was like watching a glass drop in slow motion – it was only a matter of time until it would hit the ground and shatter. All I could do was prepare myself with a vacuum cleaner to suck up all the shards.

I went to see Dr Pal, who put me on a new antidepressant, but it was hard for me to passively wait for it to work. I'd always been a 'solutions' girl, and taken an active approach to problem-solving. Allowing a drug to re-equilibrate my brain chemistry, not knowing when or how I was going to get better, was the biggest trust experiment of my life.

A few more weeks went by. It was now early October. I couldn't get out of bed most days. I didn't shower or change out of my pyjamas for days at a time – I was in bed all day and didn't sweat so I didn't see the need. Perhaps this drug wasn't going to be my Messiah.

I knew I was in a bad place. I made another appointment with Dr Pal. I was really disappointed in myself. I had done such a good thing going to Bali. I became a yoga teacher, for god's sake. Yoga teachers have their lives together. They know how to breathe and chill out. They are healthy and happy. Namaste. Yet look at me – I'm not living life as an exemplary yogi. I was an embarrassment. My recovery was not linear. It felt like I was playing a real-life version of snakes and ladders. I had been climbing steadily up a ladder but now I'd hit a snake and fallen back a few squares to a worse place than when I began.

Dr Pal was worried. She changed my antidepressants again, this time to Efexor, and gave me something else for sleep. She wanted to admit me to a nearby private hospital, but I declined. Hospital is for people who are really sick. I knew I was depressed and I knew I was tired, but I persisted in thinking I wasn't that sick.

37

Doctor becomes patient

2018, Sydney

A week passed. Things didn't get better at home. One morning
I was sitting in the middle of my apartment barely able to
move. I was wearing pyjamas that I'd put on a few days before.
I had spilled some muesli and milk on them but I couldn't be
bothered to change. My scalp was itchy and greasy because
I hadn't washed my hair. Who was this hobo I'd turned into?
Maybe it *was* time to admit myself to hospital. But there were
a few things that bothered me. I didn't want to bump into any
doctors I knew. Even though we learn psychiatry in medical
school, doctors can be harsh to each other. We accept when
patients have mental illnesses, but if it's a colleague there can
be a lot of stigma attached. It's seen as a sign of weakness or a
personality flaw. I was realising that I held the same prejudices
and I needed to fight them. I didn't want to admit to anyone,
not even myself, that I was mentally unwell. But it was time to
be honest with myself. I needed help.

I contacted Dr Pal and waved the proverbial white flag, and then I cried. I cried because I felt sorry for myself. How did things get this bad? I'm a marathon runner. I am mentally strong. Why is this happening to me, of all people? They were also tears of relief that someone was finally going to look after me. My parents still had no idea that I was even sick. They thought I was working as a Plastics registrar. I updated my sisters, explaining that I was going to be a patient for a short stint. Just three weeks, I reassured them, and then I'll be right.

Any relief I had was tempered by my dread of going to hospital. I could remember the psychiatric ward when I was a medical student. It stank. There were people screaming. It was dirty. Dr Pal reassured me that this place would be nice. She was admitting me to a private facility that had been recently built.

She was right. When I arrived, the front reception smelled like fresh detergent and was decorated with a large bouquet of flowers. I felt lucky that I had the privilege of private health insurance. I knew many others wouldn't have had the same luxury. A nurse came to pick me up, and escorted me to my room. I unpacked my things and placed some scented candles on my bedside table.

'You can't have those here,' he said, motioning me to hand them over.

'Oh, I'm sorry.' I gave him the candles.

'You can have them back when you're discharged, but I have to lock them up.'

That's when it hit me that I was officially an inpatient in a psychiatric facility. Of course, anything that could potentially be used to self-harm had to be confiscated. Part of me felt it was a bit ridiculous. Then I thought back to when I'd burned my hand earlier in the year.

It was surreal to be on the other side of the treatment equation in a hospital setting. A registrar, my doctor, assessed me, the patient, in a consultation room. She explained that the expected duration of the admission would be three weeks. She handed me a sheet of paper with the daily activity schedule.

07.30 breakfast

08.00 medications

08.30 art therapy

As someone who needed routine, I found it comforting to read the timetable. I had some blood tests and I waited.

That afternoon, the doctor returned with a consultant called Dr Aung, with whom she'd discussed me.

'There is a big element of trauma in your presentation,' Dr Aung said.

That surprised me. Being 'traumatised' made me seem like a victim; it didn't feel right.

'Your antidepressants will remain the same for now, but we'll organise for you to see a psychologist to help process the trauma you've been through.'

'Can I ask something?' I said, still not entirely accepting my diagnosis even though I'd been treated for depression for several months now. 'Do you believe in adrenal fatigue?' I was clutching at straws. *Anything but depression, please. Just give me any other diagnosis.*

'You very clearly fit the criteria for depression,' Dr Aung said firmly.

That night, I jumped at the sound of my phone ringing. Once again I had to calm myself down. *Yumiko, you're not on call, it's okay.* I looked at my phone and there was nothing there. False alarm. It was my head playing tricks on me again. There was, however, a notification that Dr Bruno had messaged me an hour ago. 'How's the article going? Can you respond to my email?' *No, Dr Bruno, I cannot.* I couldn't bear the thought of opening a Word document pinned with all of his red comment boxes. I had also received a message from Dr Whiteley, who asked if I was free to assist her in the private hospital. I told her that *I* was in hospital, and she said she would visit. I normally wouldn't have wanted visitors, but the benzos they'd put me on had made me disinhibited. It was a free-for-all. Heck, I may even have allowed Dr Sansevieria to come. Wouldn't that have been a scene.

The next morning, I woke up with a vivid, gruesome image in my head. My hands had been cut off at the wrists by a chunky pair of scissors. I decided that I would paint it during art therapy. I sat on my own, well away from the other patients because I didn't want anyone to see what I was doing. I started sketching the outline of my painting. I drew the insides of my wrist. *Flexor pollicis longus. Flexor carpi radialis.* The median nerve. My painting had to be anatomically correct – I'd been performing hand surgery for several years now, after all. This painting expressed exactly how I felt – that the hospital had metaphorically cut off my wrists so I could no longer work as a surgeon. Look at me. I'm in a psychiatric hospital and my symptoms aren't getting better. I have no idea when I'm going to be able to work again.

I dipped my brush into some red paint and tapped the brush against the table, creating a splatter of red onto my painting. Blood.

The blood tests taken on my day of admission came back that afternoon. My cholesterol was alarmingly high. I called Mariko and told her about it.

'Shit,' she said. 'That's higher than Dad's was when he had his heart attack.'

'Shit,' I echoed. But really nothing shocked me anymore. Having high cholesterol made sense to my medical brain. The stress hormone cortisol would have done that. In times of stress, the adrenal glands release cortisol, which releases glucose and fatty acids into the bloodstream to give the body more energy. My body would have had to do that for months. I knew it was disturbing for a young, previously fit person to have high cholesterol, but I was too numb to care about anything.

After a few days in the hospital I felt uncomfortable that I was there without my loved ones knowing. I needed to tell my mum. I had kept my life a secret for the past four months because I didn't want my parents to know that I'd quit my job. Maybe now I was in hospital they'd be a bit more forgiving. I hesitated a few times, but finally took the plunge and FaceTimed Yoshiko. My heart was beating so fast with every ring. She picked up and noticed immediately I wasn't at home. 'Where are you?' she asked.

'I'm in the hospital. I'm . . . I'm here as a patient, actually.'

'Oh,' was all Yoshiko could say.

'I'm kind of in a rehab-type place. I overworked myself to exhaustion, you see.'

'I see . . .' she echoed, sounding blindsided.

'So, yeah, I had to quit work. I'm not working as a registrar right now.'

Even though we were five thousand miles apart, I could read Yoshiko's face. She was gutted. She couldn't get many words out, but she told me to take it easy. It was an enormous weight off my shoulders. I wasn't quite ready to share my diagnosis with my parents, but at least they knew that I wasn't working right now.

In the second week, Dr Aung changed my medications abruptly, so I had to withdraw from Efexor. Withdrawing made me feel dreadful. I was crying for no good reason and was extremely sensitive to sights and sounds.

A few days later the nurse in charge gathered all of us in one of the common rooms. A man from our ward had gone out for a walk and got hit by a bus. He was unable to be revived by paramedics and died on the scene. He was supposed to go home the next day. He had a wife and two daughters who would have been so excited to have him back. We were told that it was an accident, but my mind went automatically to the obvious place: we are patients in a psychiatric unit. Did he deliberately walk in front of the bus? Even though I had only talked to this man a handful of times, I felt a deep sadness. Another lady was bawling. 'Just ignore me,' she said, grabbing a tissue box. 'I'm withdrawing from Efexor.'

'Same!' I called out, shocking myself by how disinhibited I was. My mood swings were wild. I was easily agitated. Even the slightest noise would bother me. It was frightening that I had no control over my emotions, and exhausting, plus I still wasn't sleeping at night despite taking a smorgasbord of sedatives. I was on a total of seven pills every day, and at night I'd ask for extra benzos every few hours whenever I found myself wide awake. Would I ever sleep a full night again?

The next day Dr Whiteley came to visit me.

'Oh, you don't look that bad,' she said. 'I thought you were going to be a lot worse.'

Once more, I didn't know how to take that. I thought maybe it was a compliment – did she mean that I was looking well? But I also knew that doctors were sceptical of other doctors' illnesses. And quite rightly so. There *were* a few who chucked dishonest sickies. I remembered a story Dr Whiteley had told me a few years before during one of her operating lists. A plastic surgeon had taken time off when his grandmother died. Except that same grandmother died three times over the course of his time as a registrar. I knew Dr Whiteley cared enough to pay me a visit at the hospital, but there was no getting away from it: her comment made me feel like she didn't believe me. It reminded me of the plastic surgeons at the hospital who hadn't taken me seriously when I asked for help. And when Neil had dismissed my chronic fatigue in medical school. How 'bad' did I have to be for people to believe that I was sick? Perhaps I looked well on the outside, but on the inside I most definitely wasn't fine.

By the end of the third week, it was clear I wouldn't be discharged. I was not responding well to the medication changes. It was frustrating, but at the same time I didn't want to go back to my apartment to have to fend for myself. The idea of doing dishes and laundry filled me with apathy.

Around this time, Heather was visiting Australia from California, and she wanted to see me and the other Australian yogis from our teaching course. I had offered to host her some weeks before, but I was still in the hospital. Heather was understanding and she too came to visit me. I was given permission to leave the ward, as long as I was supervised by a responsible adult – that person being Heather. So Heather and I went out for a vegan meal, where I tried vegan cheese for the first time. It tasted like real cheese! The next day I decided to write a blog post about it. I needed to keep myself busy, and writing made me feel productive, as well as being therapeutic.

I was enjoying the creative activities at the hospital. I had started drawing a series of ballerinas at art therapy. There was something beautiful about drawing human anatomy in dynamic movements. I also enjoyed music therapy. Another patient, Diana, was a professional singer. She had a stunning, soulful voice. It was a little raspy from all the cigarettes she smoked, but I liked its rough texture. There was something raw and authentic about it. Sometimes she and I would stay back after music class and keep singing. We harmonised to different gospel songs. I could feel the sound vibrating in my throat and down to my diaphragm. It was a comforting sensation. Having the opportunity to reconnect with the creative side of my brain was helping me more than anything else at the hospital.

When I got back to my room after singing with Diana one afternoon, there was a text message from Dr Bruno. 'Can you send back the article with the changes?' it said. *Go away.* I hadn't responded to any of his messages or emails for several months now. I was surprised he kept persisting. Maybe he was used to registrars neglecting their academic work when things got too busy at the hospital. To him, I might have been one of those registrars who needed prompting and reminding. Did he ever wonder if something could be wrong? Regardless, I continued to ignore him. I knew I was being rude, but I just couldn't cope. Part of me thought, *come on, just do it, just a few changes and I can get this thing published*. But what was the point? If I wasn't going to get back into plastic surgery – or any surgery – then an extra publication didn't mean anything.

There was still one thing I wanted to do, which was to tell Yoshiko my diagnosis. I asked myself, *if I ever have a daughter, how would I feel if she kept something like this from me?* I knew I had to tell her. So one evening I braced myself and dialled my parents' number.

'Mama,' I said nervously after we'd greeted one another.

'What is it, Yumiko?'

'I need to tell you something.'

'Okay.'

'Well, you know how I've been in here for exhaustion?'

'Yes.'

'They think the exhaustion is a symptom. A symptom of . . . depression.'

There was a pause. Then Mum said simply, 'I see.'

'I'm sorry, Mum,' I said. 'I should have told you earlier but I couldn't. You know what it's like in Japan. Mental health is still a taboo.'

'Honey,' she said. 'It's twenty-eighteen. It's not a taboo.'

As soon as I heard Yoshiko say that, I felt like I could breathe again. Keeping this from her had been weighing heavily on my heart and I was not expecting her to be so accepting. My face was hot and I could feel some tears brimming. Maybe I had underestimated my mother. I felt silly for feeling scared to tell her my truth, and it was so liberating to finally do so.

'Yumiko, come home for Christmas,' she said. 'Your family will always look after you.'

'I know,' I said. 'Thanks, Mama.'

By the sixth week, the hospital was planning my discharge, even though I didn't quite feel ready to go back home and look after myself. I'd been trialled on a new medication but it hadn't worked, so I was back on Efexor. When I got home there would be no nurses to wake me up in the morning, no organised activities to structure my day, no food prepared for me.

I was discharged on several addictive medications that were only meant to be used short term. The instructions given to my GP were just to 'wean them off'. I was also given my candles back, and my prescription. I was on my own. Holding a set of keys for the first time in six weeks felt weird, as did the motion of turning the key in the lock of my apartment, after not having lived behind a locked door for a number of weeks.

Walking inside my apartment I felt helpless. I was a little better than I'd been six weeks before, but as soon as I was alone in that space everything felt like a battle. I didn't want to cook. I resorted to eating cereal again. That night I still didn't sleep. The next morning I had cereal for breakfast.

Though I was lethargic, I was overcome by a sudden urgency to get rid of any bad juju. I decided to throw out everything in my apartment that reminded me of Medicine. I looked at the top of my bookshelf, where my loupes sat in their shiny metal box, a vestige of my microsurgery days. I decided that they could stay, but I grabbed a cardboard box and started filling it with textbooks. Talley and O'Connor. Moore and Dalley. Rang and Dale. Grabb and Smith. Why were they all white men? The books made me think of the many subconscious ways in which I was told that I had no place in a white man's world. I tossed them into the box, and then threw in my notes from the surgical primary exams. I put the box by my front door to take out with the trash.

I went to see Dr Pal two weeks after my discharge. We were both disappointed – there really wasn't much change to my overall condition. She gave me a new tablet to help me sleep.

It was nearly the end of 2018, the worst year of my life. The only saving grace was that this year I would not have to ask for annual leave to take Christmas and New Year off. And even though I was still struggling to function day to day, it was better than the hellish time I'd had at the hospital. It was such a relief not to be the on-call plastic surgery registrar, although my sleep problems relentlessly made me feel like I was still on call every night. I was looking forward to seeing my family. *I'm coming home.*

38

There's no place like home

Christmas 2018, Tokyo

When I disembarked at Narita Airport, I spotted Mariko's grinning face straightaway. The cutie was holding a 'Welcome Home' poster on which she'd drawn reindeer and snowmen. I couldn't help but have a big smile on my face as I walked over and hugged her tightly. Hajime was also on spotting duty at the entrance hall. He gave me a polite, fatherly hug. He looked a little frail, but in good spirits.

Yoshiko and Eriko were preparing dinner at my parents' apartment. When I got there, they too wrapped me in hugs. The sweet smell of mirin in the air took me back to my childhood, and I instantly felt I was home. I was safe. I took my suitcase to the tatami room, where the floor was made of woven rush and rice straw; a smell that filled me with nostalgia.

We put on the evening news. There'd been a huge blast in Sapporo as two men were emptying deodorising spray cans. Many were injured, and buildings a hundred metres away were damaged from the explosion. One of the men had serious facial burns, to which Mariko exclaimed, 'Yumiko could help him!' An innocent little remark catalysed a chain reaction of grief inside of me. No, I can't help him. I don't do plastic surgery anymore. I felt sadness in my stomach, and left the living room to let some tears out in the tatami room. I looked at my right hand. You, my little size 6, hardworking hand, have fixed many a fracture and wound. I traced the outline of the burn on the back of that hand as though it were an island floating in the sea of my skin.

Usually when I arrived in Tokyo I'd go to the park across from my parents' place, or the shops, reacquainting myself with a city that was dear to me. But the day after I flew in this time, I couldn't make my body move. I stayed in the tatami room all day, every day, like a *hikikomori* – a recluse in Japan, severely withdrawn from society. Yoshiko came in to encourage me to go visit Grandma, but I couldn't. 'Give me a few days,' I said. I also had just one request for her: 'Please, promise me, we won't talk about my job.'

I had brought my laptop with me, and I decided to begin drafting my experience of 2018 on my blog. The end of year was always a reflective time for me. Usually I'd be thinking ahead to my next clinical terms – what position I'd be taking on at which hospital, and my strategy for the Program application. This year was different. It was important for me to write everything down. Even though I wasn't sure if I was ready to write about what happened, I didn't want to leave it for too long – I knew that when people go through trauma, their brains forget certain parts of that trauma, and I didn't want to forget anything. I wasn't sure whether anyone would read my blog post, or if it would make any impact, but I needed to do it for me. I needed a record of this significant and transformative life event. So, one day before Christmas, I sat in the tatami room, cross-legged with my laptop. At first, dredging up some text, anything, was really hard. As soon as I began, the idea of recapping the four months of hell at that south-west Sydney hospital filled me with dread and disgust. I wrote for about an hour, and then I gave up.

Within a few days of being in Tokyo, I realised that the visit was helping me more than my stint at the private hospital had. No matter how much I trusted science and medicine and doctors, there was no healer more powerful than a mother's love. Yoshiko's care was soothing, like Manuka honey. She knew all of my favourite Japanese dishes. The familiar aroma of her wonderful cooking danced in my nose. At night, she would tuck me under a huge doona, which we call *kakebutons*. In the mornings, she'd gently come to wake me up with a hot coffee – it was comfort in a mug. She knew not to push me when I was simply feeling too weak, but on my better days she'd encourage me to go for a walk with Grandma.

On Christmas Day I received the best gift of all: sleep. After exchanging presents with my sisters, I went back to sleep and I did not get up until Boxing Day. It wasn't exactly uninterrupted, but I had a few solid blocks of luxurious, deep, restorative sleep, as though I were sinking to the bottom of the ocean, insulated from any sounds on Earth. The new sleeping tablet that Dr Pal had prescribed seemed to be working, and I think there was something about the *kakebutons*. They were much heavier than normal doonas, like weighted blankets.

When I woke up on Boxing Day, I was ready to do some more writing. I tapped away at the keyboard, gaining momentum as the memories came back like water released from a dam. I was surprised by how quickly and vividly I could remember some of the incidents, as they travelled through my fingertips and onto the screen. I wrote the post as though I was writing a report, so I could feel distanced from it; that it wasn't about me. I called the blog post 'The Ugly Side of Becoming a Surgeon'. There were just eleven subscribers to my blog, consisting of my family and a few friends. I didn't really care if no one read it, though, because posting was a cathartic exercise for me.

A few days before returning to Sydney, Hajime spoke to me. I had been avoiding the topic of work with him, but it was inevitable that he'd say something before the visit was over.

'Yumiko, I was thinking about your career,' he started.

I wasn't ready to be told to get back to work. I didn't want any pressure from anyone, let alone my father.

'Dad,' I interrupted, 'I'm not ready to go back to the hospital system.' I felt triggered, but I kept my cool and tried not to burst into tears.

'No, no, I'm not suggesting that at all.'

'Oh. What were you thinking, then?'

'Well, you used to love anatomy. When you taught it while you were still at medical school, you'd come home beaming! You were on such a high after every class you taught,' he said. 'Why don't you contact one of your professors? Maybe they'll give you a job.'

I was stunned. I thought Hajime would be disappointed in me for giving up surgery after being such a fervent supporter of mine. He'd always told me that I could do anything I wanted to do. He'd helped me with my university fees, as well as some textbooks and courses. I knew that part of why I had resisted telling my parents about my resignation for so long was out of guilt for all the financial and moral support they'd given me over the years. But Hajime didn't make me feel bad about any of it. He was very encouraging about me finding a new career path in academia.

'You've worked so hard,' he said. 'Too hard, in fact. Don't break your body.'

'Thanks, Dad.' I felt a little lump in my throat.

His words seemed carefully chosen. *Don't break your body.* I wondered whether this was always how my father would have responded to such situations, or whether having had a massive heart attack followed by cancer had changed his view on life. The physical traumas that Hajime had gone through in the last few years were a sobering lesson to all of us.

39

Kintsugi

2019, Sydney

Back in Sydney, Maxence invited me to a dinner with some surgeons and medical students. I hadn't been to any dinners for several months because I had been so socially withdrawn, and I especially didn't want to see anyone related to the medical field. Now, I felt different. I thought I was going to be okay interacting with medical people.

Max introduced me to Dr Shaw, a plastic surgeon visiting from Queensland.

'Oh, what an exotic dress,' said Dr Shaw. 'You look like Lee Lin Chin.'

'Thank you,' I said. I was a fan of the treasured newsreader, but I couldn't help but feel the racial undertones.

'Let me buy you a drink,' he said, looking at the drinks menu. 'My Asian housekeeper tells me that you people like aloe vera. How about this one?' he asked, pointing at Aloe Sailor, a yuzu-flavoured cocktail.

366

'That sounds lovely,' I said politely, immediately cross with myself for validating his stereotype.

'Waitress!' he called out at a member of staff walking by. 'Two Aloe Sailors.'

'Two Aloe Sailors,' she repeated and jotted down in her notebook.

'One for me, one for Lee Lin Chin,' he said, chortling at his own joke.

On my end of the table was a young medical student, Madison, who was interested in becoming a surgeon. Dr Shaw was giving her his two cents.

'You need to do research,' he said. 'What sort of surgery do you want to do?'

'Plastics,' she said. I tried to look excited for her. Inside I was squirming.

'Very good,' said Dr Shaw. 'You want a research project?'

'Yes, please,' she said, eager-eyed.

'I'll hook you up,' he said, with a confident smirk.

'Oh, thank you so much!' she exclaimed.

I couldn't bear this conversation. This poor girl was only in second-year medical school; she had hardly spent a hot minute on the wards. She had no idea. I felt conflicted. I genuinely wanted to support my younger colleagues and their career aspirations. But after everything I'd been through, I also felt a sense of responsibility. Enter at your own risk. The more Dr Shaw spoke about how Maddy could improve her CV, the more my heart pounded. She reminded me of how bright-eyed and bushy-tailed I was at that stage of my life. I would have been eighteen years old as a second-year student. I wasn't jaded or cynical, as I was now. I was ready and willing to do anything to succeed in surgery. Seeing the stars in Madison's eyes crushed me. I excused myself and walked down a spiral staircase to the bathrooms. I locked myself in a cubicle and cried. Maybe I wasn't ready to hang out with doctors and medical students.

I returned to the other end of the table and drew an extra chair over to sit next to Maxence.

'I can't be here, Max,' I said, shaking.

'What? What's wrong, Yumes?' he asked.

'Dr Shaw is giving career advice to Madison,' I said. 'It's killing me. It's bringing back some stuff.'

'Oh, Yumes, just sit on this end of the table for a little bit. We're talking about astrophysics,' he said. That made me laugh.

'I'm on another planet,' I said. 'I have no idea about physics.'

'How about some dessert?'

'That always makes me feel better,' I said. 'Let's get the cheesecake.'

I didn't sleep that night. All I could think about was the look on Maddy's face – so enthralled. I wondered how many years she'd spend working in a hospital before realising that it wasn't as glamorous as it might seem.

It was nearly February. I should have been starting a new clinical year but I remained too mentally unwell to work. The trip to Japan had helped me recover some strength, and I was sleeping better, but I couldn't help thinking back to Dr Perera's prediction: that she couldn't see me back to any hospital environment for at least a year.

I thought about my father's suggestion and emailed my former anatomy professor. A response came straightaway.

'We'd love to have you back,' he said. He had stepped down from his role as the head of Anatomy, and copied in Professor Pillay to the emails. Professor Pillay was a South African-born Indian-Australian woman. I was surprised and impressed to see a woman of colour at the helm of the department. In all my time as a student and junior doctor, I had never seen that. It made me reflect on how much diversity there was in the medical student cohort that didn't translate to higher positions. I wondered what the new cohort of interns looked like, who were starting at hospitals around Australia in the first week of February. My thoughts moved to all the unaccredited registrars beginning a new year, and the pressure on them to get good references for this year's application to the Program.

I went back to the blog I'd written in Japan: 'The Ugly Side of Becoming a Surgeon'. I reread it and suddenly felt an urge to share it with more readers. My family and friends had been supportive of the article, but I knew it was something the medical community needed to read. It was important. The toxic culture was driving out so many doctors, and in some cases driving them even to death, as I thought about Charlie's cousin, Loy.

I decided to get in touch with a friend I'd gone to medical school with who was now involved heavily in the Australian Medical Association. I wasn't really sure what it would achieve, but I guess I just wanted someone important to read it and make me feel seen. I thought maybe she'd care about my story since the AMA did so much work advocating for doctors.

'Sure, send it to my AMA email,' she said.

Days went by and she hadn't responded. And so, on Sunday the third of February, the day before the new clinical year was to begin for all junior doctors in Australia, I posted my blog to Facebook with the relevant hashtags. I also tagged RACS and the AMA. *Thank you, Bev, I finally have some use for all the SEO training you made me do for your website.* I wondered whether SEO really worked. Would anyone read this?

Within a few hours, I started receiving comments. Some simply tagged other users, sometimes with a remark like 'This is so sad.' Others addressed me directly to say 'Sorry that happened to you,' or 'Thanks for writing this.' Some people had their own personal stories to share, and these started to fill my inbox. I heard from former colleagues, including some residents from the hospital who said they had no idea I was burned out because I'd appeared cheerful to them. I even heard from an ED consultant there, thanking me for being nice to work with despite what I was going through at the time. An intern messaged me to say that I had taught a few of her friends when they were medical students, who had no clue I was having it tough because I had taught them with such enthusiasm and generosity. She also mentioned that I had turned around a couple of her friends who'd had serious thoughts about leaving Medicine. I dwelled on that particular message for a long time. How was I able to encourage others to love Medicine, when I myself was so heartbroken?

Doctors, nurses and allied health professionals from all around the world sent heartfelt messages. I even heard from their parents, siblings and partners, who would have suffered just as much, if not more, watching their loved ones burn to the ground.

Burnout, I realised, was a universal phenomenon. It was incredible that these strangers felt they could confide in me about their situations. Some of them wrote paragraphs and paragraphs. Many said they'd cried when they read my blog post.

I couldn't stop looking at my phone. I clicked on the little bell icon on Facebook every few minutes to refresh my notifications. I couldn't eat. Before I knew it, it was well past midnight and there were a hundred private messages unread. The little red number on my Instagram app alerted me to messages that were coming in there, too.

The next day, I was contacted by Kate Aubusson, a journalist from the *Sydney Morning Herald*. Whoa. I wasn't expecting it to reach the mainstream media. How had my little blog of eleven subscribers reached her? The idea of speaking to her made me a bit nervous. I hadn't dealt with the media before – it's something most doctors shy away from. I was worried about coming across unfavourably and on top of all the mental health problems I already had, I didn't want to get trolled. I did, however, know that Kate had an excellent reputation as an investigative journalist among the medical community.

We spoke on the phone for an hour or so. She was empathetic and kind, and treated our conversation with sensitivity. That afternoon, a photographer came to my apartment to take photos for the newspaper. It was all happening so quickly. It felt amazing to finally be heard, and to have so many others coming forth saying they could relate. At the same time, it was quite stressful. Now that there was a bit of public attention, I felt I needed to be careful about every word I said. I didn't want to say the wrong thing because I knew I'd be scrutinised. I felt pressured to answer every message I received, so that the people who'd spent their time writing me a message didn't feel snubbed. I spent hours replying to people, making sure that I was thoughtful and empathetic in my response to them.

For my photo for the paper, I decided to wear a simple crocheted gold dress, which was symbolic to me. In Japan, *kintsugi* means to 'join with gold'. It's a method of repairing broken pottery with lacquer powdered with gold. The gold fractures are celebrated rather than concealed, and considered a unique part of the object's history. There I was, in my gold dress, like *kintsugi* holding me together, fractured for all to see, but stronger and more beautiful because of the pain I'd been through. Kate called the article, 'Exhausted Surgeon Dismissed as "Emotional Female"'.

The article became the number one trending piece on the *Sydney Morning Herald* website when it was published. The next day, it went to print. Doctors I hadn't spoken to in years were coming out as my 'friends' and commenting on online forums and social media. My AMA contact, from whom I'd heard nothing since I'd emailed her my blog post, was on the television screen speaking to a news reporter about how brave I was. Those with political megaphones were virtue-signalling, engaging in online threads about the issues that had been raised in my blog post. None of them had reached out to me directly to check that I was okay. Some of it felt performative.

I realised that it wasn't about me anymore. My post was something I'd written for myself in the small confines of the tatami room in Tokyo, to document the worst time of my life. But now it had almost instantly become a conduit for medico-political discussion. Issues I hadn't even thought about explicitly, or in the terms they were being talked about, were highlighted: burnout, mental health, bullying and harassment in the workplace, exploitation of junior doctors, and the micro-aggressions and unconscious bias against women – especially those of colour – in the medical profession. In a strange way, even though I had written the blog post, I was learning from it, too. I hadn't used the term 'microaggression' before, for example. I had spent the past fifteen years of my life studying clinical sciences, so this was an opportunity for me to educate myself on the social sciences and become a better advocate for others like me.

The media furore over the next few days was a blur. I was trying hard to answer requests for interviews from television, radio, podcasts, and magazines from around the world. I was talking to people from countries as far away as Poland and Colombia. Over the past decade, there had been plenty of reports by senior doctors, researchers and academics about burnout and bullying in Medicine. However, without a human face, the numbers blend into the background, making it easy to dismiss such incidents as things that happened to other people. It was rare for a doctor, and especially a junior doctor, to put their name and face out into the blogosphere, or any -sphere for that matter, with their personal story. I was starting to realise the power of shared, lived experience. Doctors tend to be private creatures, and there is a professional code of silence where we don't complain about our jobs, even when the things that are happening are unacceptable, or illegal even – Caroline Tan being an example of what can happen to you if you speak up. So, we just shut up and get on with it. There's too much at stake. If I were still aspiring to get on to the Program, there's no way I would have blogged about my experiences. I could only do it because I had nothing to lose. And perhaps the benzos I was on made me disinhibited. No fucks given. I had become the voice for all the junior doctors who were muzzled by the system.

Now that the blog post had garnered mainstream interest, the colleges, medical associations and health departments had some addressing to do. An email arrived from Medical Services at the south-west Sydney hospital inviting me to have a conversation with them about how to make things better for junior doctors. Never mind the multiple attempts I'd made nearly a year ago to have this very discussion. The letter closed by saying they thought that after I'd left the hospital, I'd gone back 'home' to Japan, otherwise they would have contacted me sooner. Everything about that statement encapsulated the attitudes I'd come across there: casual racism, a hefty dose of complacency, and another dose of negligence when it came to their duty of care to staff their systems had harmed.

I also received a message from a representative of RACS. 'The College can pay for some counselling,' she said. I almost laughed when I read that. As an unaccredited registrar, I hadn't fallen under their responsibility, and now I wished they'd kept it that way rather than suggest that all I needed was 'some counselling'. It was so insulting. Why not address the lack of institutional leadership shown by my bosses – fellows of RACS – that had led to my poor treatment?

EPILOGUE

Petrichor

December 2019, Sydney

Petrichor is that glorious, damp smell of rain on earth after a long dry spell. One December morning at the end of 2019, I got up, walked to my kitchen and made myself a cup of coffee. As I was pouring the milk from the frother, I took in a deep breath and enjoyed the aroma of the coffee. I felt strangely alert. It usually took me a bit longer to wake up, but I felt fresh. And then I thought to myself, *did I just sleep the whole night? I did, I think I really did.* I just had my first full night of sleep in eighteen months. Was I *finally* emancipated from the shackles of insomnia? I was overwhelmed with relief and gratitude. I hugged my cup between my hands, and wept. Petrichor. That was the smell of my first deep sleep.

The other symptoms of my depression had also eased. I was feeling more energetic. I had reconnected with friends, my circle, and felt less social anxiety. I was able to enjoy things like yoga, the beach or, even better, yoga on the beach. I wasn't relying on prescription pills to make me sleep, although I had grown to accept medications. I told myself that if I needed to take tablets to function, then that's what I needed, and that's okay. I never thought that I would suffer from a mental illness, but I did, and maybe it had happened to me for a reason. *Isvara pranidhana*. Surrender to the universe. I allowed myself to heal in my own time, and I learned to accept myself in whatever state of suffering I was in. My mental illness had a precipitant that I knew to avoid in the future: being overworked. My health comes first. I will never allow myself to be treated like that again. I need to set boundaries, and learn to say 'no'. I give myself permission to live a calm and happy life.

My life was looking different, but different was just fine by me. For the longest time, I was searching for the perfect mentor and role model, but what I realised was that those people don't exist. Maybe finding this unicorn was unrealistic. There were female physicians like Professor Bloom, and male surgeons like Dr Stein, to whom I looked up, but there weren't many female surgeons. I'd worked with Bernadette, Dr Whiteley and Dr Sansevieria, representing three generations of female plastic surgeons, but modelling myself after them didn't feel right. This was part of the problem for women in surgery – the lack of visible role models. We all have different values, priorities and goals in life, so this notion of using someone 'better' and more 'successful' than myself as a cookie cutter was flawed. What does success mean anyway? I had encountered many successful surgeons who were unhappy. I realised that we had to become our own role models and lead a life that we find worth living, and that's something only you yourself can do.

It was nearly Christmas again, and I was thankful that I was able, once more, to go to Japan to be with my family during this special time of year. I was a different person to the Yumiko of a year ago. As I flew to Tokyo I reflected on what had happened in 2019. The year had not at all been what I had expected. My blog post had reached about 200,000 views. At the institutional level it had become a part of the curriculum at medical schools that teach students about burnout. The AMA in New South Wales had released a statement called 'Protections for doctors-in-training' in response to my post, saying: '[Kadota's] experiences and the subsequent reaction from within medicine highlighted the need for change. The Doctors-in-Training Committee (DITC) has been a strong advocate for better support from the health system and continues to lobby for greater protections for both unaccredited and accredited registrars.'

It makes me feel good knowing that I have, at least in small part, contributed towards a dialogue to change how junior doctors are treated. I am, however, aware that statements do not necessarily translate to action. There is so much to discuss in this sphere. The medical profession has put – had already put – measures into place to try to address the issues I experienced and that many of my colleagues are still enduring. Whether these measures are effective is another matter, so we need to keep debating and questioning their efficacy. It takes more than policy changes, no matter how well meant or seemingly radical, to lead to real, cultural shifts.

Nothing can take away what happened to me. Those few years will always remain a part of my life where my physical, mental, and spiritual health suffered. But I wanted – and continue to want – to talk about them with anyone who may benefit from what I went through. In 2019, that's what I did. I travelled around Australia to connect with students, doctors, and allied health professionals to tell them about my experiences.

People drew from my blog what they needed to. For fellow unaccredited registrars, the post helped them to feel seen. It gave some the courage to leave their own toxic workplaces. Others related to being a woman of colour working in a field dominated by white men. Cultural changes in large organisations don't happen overnight, but they start with small conversations. People were talking about topics like mental health, which were far more taboo in the past. The medical profession is one of the most at-risk in terms of mental illness. We know from a national survey by Beyond Blue in 2013 that one in five doctors have had a diagnosis of depression or received treatment for it. Both doctors and medical students have higher rates of psychological distress and suicidal thoughts compared to the general population, and the rates are even higher among female doctors aged thirty or younger. Young female doctors scored the highest in all three domains of burnout that were assessed: emotional exhaustion, cynicism and feeling a lack of professional achievement. Troublingly, 40 per cent of doctors felt that their peers with psychiatric diagnoses were perceived as less competent; and nearly half felt that doctors were less likely to be appointed if they had a history of mental illness. It's clear that there is still some destigmatising to do.

However, there have been some changes to the way in which we talk about burnout, which are promising. Whereas in the past, we spoke about things like individual resilience, we now know that this is an occupational phenomenon that requires institutional leadership and responsibility. 'Moral injury' has been proposed as a much better term to describe what is happening to doctors. Semantics aside, I welcomed the shift from blaming the individual to looking at systemic factors. The canary in the coalmine. The solution is not to make stronger canaries.

I started to work part-time again in May, having accepted an appointment as a lecturer in Anatomy. I remember walking into Professor Pillay's office at my alma mater. I hadn't met her before so I didn't know what to expect, although I'd heard that she was very popular among the students for being warm, approachable, and of course a fantastic teacher. As a woman of colour, I knew she would have had to work astronomically hard to make it to professorial level, and even harder to become the head of department. Was she one of those women who had smashed the glass ceiling and believed in empowering younger women to do the same? Or was she more like Dr Sansevieria, and would expect those who came after her to battle on their own, as she no doubt had?

Prof Pillay invited me to sit down. I noticed a row of thriving plants along her brightly lit windowsill. There was a croton with vibrant red and orange foliage, a philodendron pink princess and a peace lily with a few white flowers in bloom.

'I've heard a few things,' she said. 'But I want to hear it from you.'

So, she let me talk. She listened attentively and empathetically. I was honest with her when I told her that it had broken my heart to leave surgery, but I wanted her to know that I was committed to this career change.

'I loved teaching in the past, and I know I will love it again,' I said.

'I know you will,' she said. 'Your clinical experience will be valuable to the students.'

I told her how passionate I was about making anatomy interesting and relevant to medical students.

'I'm sad about what happened to you,' she said. 'But I'm here to help you rebuild a new career.'

Then, I drew a nervous breath and decided to tell Prof Pillay that I had depression. I admitted to her that I didn't have the stamina I had before, and my fear was burning out again. I felt so vulnerable and exposed, sharing that piece of myself. In the past, there's no way I would've done that. I myself took time to accept the diagnosis. But in the preceding year I had learned to be self-compassionate, and that meant setting boundaries. I wasn't going to allow myself to burn out again.

How does any one of us know who we can and cannot trust? There are invisible biases everywhere, and sometimes all you can do is put yourself out there and trust your gut. But I had a sense I could trust Prof Pillay. My gut feeling was that she wouldn't mirror the fifty per cent of my profession who might deny doctors a job because of mental health issues.

'It's okay,' she said, looking straight into my eyes. 'You tell me how much or how little you want to work. When you get better, I can give you more hours, you just let me know.'

I was surprised. Then relieved. Then so, so grateful. Here we were, two emotional females sitting opposite each other.

I felt supported and understood. When I'm in the company of an emotionally intelligent woman, it allows me to be unapologetically myself, and it reminds me that being emotional is a wonderful thing.

On my first day of teaching, there was a small cake box for me. On it, Professor Pillay had written a message with a whiteboard marker: 'Because this week might be hard for you.'

I may have given up surgery, but I am still a doctor. And I get to educate and nurture the next generation of doctors. I think I'm going to be all right.

POSTSCRIPT

I am grateful to all the readers of *Emotional Female* who have got in touch with me since the first edition was published, some of whom I've had the joy of meeting in person at various events, including the Sydney Writers' Festival (where I tried stand-up comedy for the first time in my life!).

It saddens me that some of the toxic situations I described in the book are ongoing in the public hospital system; however, I feel buoyed by fellow doctors who are also passionate about creating systemic change. As well as fellow women – especially women of colour – in Medicine who could relate to my story, I have also heard from the leadership at the Royal Australasian College of Surgeons and the Australian Society of Plastic Surgeons.

The COVID pandemic has meant I have been separated from my family members, who all live in Tokyo, for more months than I care to think about. They are all doing well, including my father, Hajime, who has been in remission from lymphoma.

I have been able to return to clinical work since the first edition of my book came out. Three plastic surgeons in Sydney have taken me under their wing and I work as their assistant surgeon in the operating theatres. I am also working in private practice as a cosmetic physician. I am still too traumatised to return to any sort of public hospital work. Mental-health-wise, it has taken me more than three years to recover from burnout and depression. Doing resistance exercise was something my psychiatrist recommended and I now teach Body Pump classes around Sydney, which I absolutely love. I also intend to undertake a third yoga teacher training course. I continue to feel grateful for how much yoga has improved my way of living.

ACKNOWLEDGEMENTS

I have a big tribe of emotional females to thank for helping me to bring this book to life!

First, I must thank my agent, Clare Forster from Curtis Brown. At the start of 2019, when my blog post first hit the news, I had no idea what a literary agent even was. Thank you, Clare, for all the hand-holding, introducing me to the world of publishers, and getting me in touch with the wonderful women at Penguin Random House!

Big thank you to my publisher, Nikki Christer. From the moment I met Nikki, I knew she was fully invested in my story. Thank you for being so generous with your time, making sure I was okay during the writing process, and being so encouraging even when I didn't have confidence in my ability to write this book.

To Roberta Ivers, who helped me with the first structural edit – thank you. I learned so much from you. It was a steep learning curve, having never written a memoir before. Your technical expertise, honesty and passion really helped me elevate this book.

To Catherine Hill – thank you for all the hard work you put into the editing process. From the first time I met you, I knew I could trust you. I felt we had a similar taste in writing, and that you would treat the book with great care and respect. Thank you for being so thoughtful. I will really miss seeing your name in my inbox!

Thanks to every single person from Penguin Random House who has worked to get my story out there. I honestly feel as though each member of the team was behind me from the start, even before we met in person. I know that a lot of work goes on behind the scenes at different stages. I'm so grateful for the incredible support and enthusiasm for this book from all departments.

To everyone who had my back during some of the toughest times in my career – thank you. I remember the small acts of kindness. All of them. It's sad that I wasn't able to continue, but I look back fondly at some of the years I spent as a doctor in the public health system, and all the friendships I made.

Thank you to my GP and psychiatrist for looking after me when I was so, so unwell. Being a doctor can be a thankless job, but I hope you know how much I appreciate everything you've done for me to help me get back to good health. It's taken a very long time, but I always had faith that you'd get me through it and I won't forget your kind words. Thank you, from the bottom of my heart.

A special thank you to my sisters, to whom this book is dedicated. You've always been my unwavering cheer squad. When times were low, you sent so many BuzzFeed quizzes to help me figure out what sort of potato I was, based on my personality traits (I'm a waffle fry). Even though you're both in Japan now, our group chat always keeps me going. I'm so lucky to have sisters as best friends. I'm proud of you, and love you both.

Last but not least, many thanks to you – my reader – for picking up this book. Perhaps 'enjoy' is the wrong word, given some of the difficult content in here, but I hope it was worth the read. Thank you for giving up your time to read my story.

Yumiko Kadota is a medical doctor who lives in Sydney. She left the public hospital system in 2018 due to burnout and a toxic work environment. A blog post she wrote on this topic entered the mainstream media in early 2019 and led to the opportunity to write this book. Yumiko now writes and speaks about her experiences on various platforms – you can catch interviews with her on Mamamia No Filter with Mia Freedman, Shameless, Better Reading, and the Booktopia podcast. She has also spoken at events such as the Leadership Summit by Future Women.

mindbodymiko.com

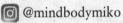 @mindbodymiko

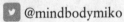 @mindbodymiko

Discover a
new favourite

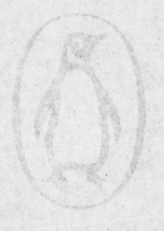

Discover a
new favourite